Living Well with a Serious Illness

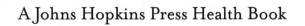
A Johns Hopkins Press Health Book

Living Well

with a

Serious Illness

A Guide to Palliative Care
for Mind, Body, and Spirit

ROBIN BENNETT KANAREK

JOHNS HOPKINS UNIVERSITY PRESS
Baltimore

Note to the reader: This book is not meant to substitute for medical care, and treatment should not be based solely on its contents. Instead, treatment must be developed in a dialogue between the individual and their physician. The book has been written to help with that dialogue.

Johns Hopkins University Press
2715 North Charles Street
Baltimore, Maryland 21218
www.press.jhu.edu

Library of Congress Cataloging-in-Publication Data is available.

ISBN 978-1-4214-4571-7 (hardcover)
ISBN 978-1-4214-4598-4 (paperback)
ISBN 978-1-4214-4572-4 (ebook)

A catalog record for this book is available from the British Library.

Jan Kochanowski's poem "On Health," translated by Jarek Zawadzki, is licensed under CC BY-SA 3.0 (page vii). Clare Harner's poem "Immortality" is from the December 1934 edition of *The Gypsy* (chapter 8).

Special discounts are available for bulk purchases of this book. For more information, please contact Special Sales at specialsales@jh.edu.

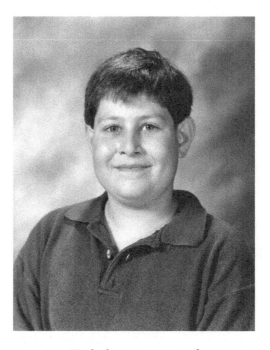

To the loving memory of

David Bennett Kanarek (1984–2000).

In the body of this boy lived a man

whose courage, kindness, and

sense of humor will always inspire us.

This book is for you.

On Health
Jan Kochanowski, 1530–1584

My good and noble health,
Thou matter'st more than wealth.
None know'th thy worth until
Thou fad'st, and we fall ill.

And every man can see,
In stark reality,
And every man will say:
" 'Tis health I need today."

No better thing we know,
No dearer gem we owe,
For all that we possess:
Pearls, stones of great finesse,
High offices and power
—One may enjoy this hour—
And so the gifts of youth,
And beauty are, in truth,
Good things, but only when
Our health is with us then.
For when the body's weak,
The world around is bleak.
O jewel dear, my home
Awaiteth thee to come;
With thee it shall not perish.
'Tis all for thee to cherish.

Contents

Living Well with a Serious Illness

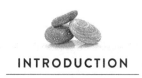

David's Story

*In the depth of winter, I finally learned that within me
there lay an invincible summer.*

—ALBERT CAMUS (1913-1960), FRENCH PHILOSOPHER,
AUTHOR, JOURNALIST, AND 1957 NOBEL PRIZE WINNER IN LITERATURE

My husband and I sat in the doctor's office, anxiously awaiting an explanation about why our fifteen-year-old son was having trouble walking.

It was the summer after David had graduated from eighth grade. We'd agreed to his request to attend sleepaway camp— a significant milestone in the life of an adolescent. David was thrilled at the prospect of adventure, time with boys his own age, and a little independence.

About two weeks into David's stay at camp, one of the counselors called to tell us that David was limping and complaining about pain in his hip. We got on the phone with David, and his description of his symptoms convinced us that we had to bring him home right away. He was inconsolable; he wanted to be a normal kid doing all the fun things his campmates were doing as they enjoyed the fleeting weeks before they started their first year of high school.

Our hearts sank as we saw David limping toward us from the airport's arrival gate; we had seen that limp before, and it evoked sheer terror in us. Without telling each other until much later, Joe and I were experiencing the same reaction: we were filled with dread.

Still, we held on to hope as we sat together in the doctor's office that sun-washed afternoon, waiting for an explanation of David's symptoms. David would not be joining us for the meeting because he was still asleep from his sedation for a bone marrow aspiration that morning.

"The pathology report isn't good," the doctor said as he stepped into the room. "David's cancer is back." He paused. "It's much more aggressive this time."

The anxiety that gripped us was visceral. Still, we had been down this road before. We would get through this; David would be well again.

Four years earlier, when David, our firstborn, was a happy, seemingly healthy ten-year-old boy, he fell while roughhousing with his sister. A week later, he couldn't walk. How had such a seemingly benign activity resulted in an excruciating pain that only grew worse by the day? His pediatrician conducted a battery of tests but could find nothing wrong. Then a CT scan revealed an enlarged spleen. "I think you need to see a specialist," the doctor said. Soon after, a bone marrow aspiration gave us the devastating diagnosis: David had leukemia—specifically, acute lymphocytic leukemia, or ALL.

As with any family facing a serious, life-threatening diagnosis, our reaction was fear, disbelief, an urgent need to find answers, and a fierce desire to "fix" the problem. Modern medicine—bring it on. There was no limit to what we would do to return our ten-year-old son to good health. That also meant there would be no limit to what David would endure, but he was up for it. He wanted to live. We were prepared to pursue every medical option to make that happen, and we did.

"This is treatable. I can arrest this disease," our pediatric oncologist reassured us. "My colleagues and I have discussed David's case, and we are very optimistic. We are going to get this in remission." She was true to her word: within three weeks of undergoing intense chemotherapy, David was in remission.

"You can relax now," our well-meaning friends said when they heard the good news. But the truth is, Joe and I never relaxed. We carried on. Still, as the years went by, our family life resembled that of any working couple with two young kids. We were busy, hopeful, happy. At David's bar mitzvah, we had every indication that he was on the road to being cured. We were going to be one of the lucky families.

Now, we needed to be "lucky" again. Just as we had four years earlier, when David was first diagnosed with leukemia, we responded with a fierce intention to "fix" the problem. Yes, things were more dire this time around, but we had access to excellent medical care. We steeled ourselves for what lay ahead, knowing it would be difficult for our entire family—and most of all for David—but hopeful that, once again, modern medicine would save our son.

We returned to a routine of visits to specialists, more tests, and consideration of treatment plans. As it had before, strategizing about beating the disease consumed our days. We were told that a stem cell transplant was the best option for David, but none of us—not his father, not his sister, not I—was a perfect match. David's sister, Sarah, however, was a *close* match. The doctors explained that trying T-cell depletion before transplanting Sarah's stem cells (a relatively new procedure at the time) might mean that David's body would accept them. If all went according to the best-case scenario, Sarah's stem cells would become David's new immune system and bring him back to health.

Getting ready for a stem cell transplant is a long, arduous, and painful ordeal. David underwent chemotherapy and radiation to eradicate his immune system so that it would not attack the new stem cells. That process left him dangerously vulnerable to infections. During this time, and for weeks after the transplant, David was kept in strict isolation to protect him from exposure to germs until his new immune system was intact.

Visitors of any kind were discouraged, and health care providers entered his room only when necessary, for the briefest possible time, and only after an intense hand-washing regimen, followed by the donning of a gown, gloves, a mask, and booties. David's isolation lasted for twenty eight days. The experi ence of being quarantined had a profound effect on his state of mind. He became angry and aggressive. This dramatic change was *not* the result of his illness or the drugs he was being given; it was a direct result of his being kept apart from others, unable to experience human contact.

My husband and I began to realize that no one was paying any attention to David's psychological, social, or spiritual needs. As his mother and as a nurse, I sensed that he had questions about his mortality, but he would not allow us to broach the subject. We asked his nurses and doctors to step in, but no one felt comfortable doing so. Our experience was not unique. As Atul Gawande, a vocal proponent of palliative care (surgeon, writer, and public health researcher at Brigham and Women's Hospital, Boston), noted adamantly in a 2016 testimony before the US Senate Special Committee on Aging, "The clinical community lacks adequate skills in serious illness communication and palliative care."

Finally, we pleaded with David's favorite transplant doctor to have "the conversation." After agreeing reluctantly, he emerged from David's room three hours later. He appeared utterly exhausted from the emotionally charged exchange; all he would say before heading down the hall was "He had a lot of philosophical questions."

To our surprise, David was not depressed by their discussion. Quite the opposite, in fact—he appeared relieved and relaxed. For the first time in a long time, he was flashing his famous bright smile.

We marveled at how a doctor-patient interaction that did not involve the administration of a drug, the checking of vital signs, or a query about pain on a scale of zero to ten had such a beneficial effect. The simple act of one human being connecting with another, a doctor viewing a patient as a whole person while listening, asking, sharing, and being an honest witness for David's concerns, provided something no drug ever could. In hindsight, we recognized what Dr. Gawande was talking about in his groundbreaking book, *Being Mortal*, when he wrote, "And in a war that you cannot win, you don't want a general who fights to the point of total annihilation. You don't want Custer. You want Robert E. Lee, someone who knows how to fight for territory that can be won and how to surrender it when it can't, someone who understands that the damage is greatest if all you do is battle to the bitter end."[1]

OUR BELOVED SON'S JOURNEY ended in 2000. He was fifteen years old. Our journey has continued, beginning with our attempt to make sense of what had happened, to heal in the midst of our profound grief, and to keep our family intact. A pivotal experience in this undertaking for me early on was reading Viktor Frankl's book *Man's Search for Meaning*, in which he describes his time as a prisoner in World War II Nazi concentration camps and his work as a psychiatrist to uncover the proverbial meaning of life. I remembered that when David was going through chemo, I kept thinking about concentration camps, as the treatment process often leaves patients feeling dehumanized in a parallel way. My takeaway from Frankl's story was that even if you are under great duress and are facing a very difficult situation, you have to find the inner strength to move forward. That is what David did and what my family continues to try to do to this day.

Four months after David's death, we moved to London. I spent the next two years in grief counseling and focusing on my daughter and my husband. Eventually, I wanted to help others by sharing what I had learned from my family's experience.

I soon became involved with the Teenage Cancer Trust, a UK organization that had a unique perspective on adolescent oncology and that had built inpatient cancer units specifically for teenagers and young adults. I wanted to volunteer and use my experience as David's mom to offer support to other parents of teens with cancer.

Seven years later, back in the United States, I returned to Fairfield University in Connecticut, my alma mater, with the goal of continuing that type of work. It was there that a pediatric nurse faculty member introduced me to the concept of palliative care. I learned about palliative care teams working in pediatric oncology: doctors, advanced-practice nurses, psychologists, social workers, and chaplains collaborated through the trajectory of a patient's illness, addressing pain management, the side effects of treatment, psychosocial needs, and spiritual care. They were a rock-solid source of information and guidance, there to help the patient and their family understand choices, decipher priorities, and ensure continuity of care based on the patient's and their family's decisions.

I was intrigued by what I learned, and more than a little sad that palliative care had not been part of the treatment offered to David and our family. The unrelenting battle to eliminate his disease, regardless of the prognosis, had completely overlooked and severely limited his quality of life.

Then, in 2009, I read a front-page article in the *New York Times* in which the author, Anemona Hartocollis, implied that palliative care was one-dimensional—for hospice patients only. That prompted me to write an article for the *American Journal of Nursing* entitled "Palliative Care Isn't Just for the Dying." I explained, "In a letter to the editor published in the *New York Times* on August 29, 2009 [responding to the Hartocollis piece], Gail Austin Cooney, MD, the president of the American Academy of Hospice and Palliative Medicine, noted that palliative care 'can help patients who will live years after they receive a diagnosis of a life-threatening or chronic illness. . . . [It] can help patients better tolerate treatments as they recover.' " Dr. Cooney's letter noted that although the Hartocollis piece was detailed and sensitive in nature, it could leave the impression that palliative care is only for dying patients. Cooney further clarified that palliative care can help patients better tolerate treatment as they recuperate. All of this transpired right before I started thinking really differently about palliative care and served as the impetus for writing this book.

I reached another tipping point in my advocacy for palliative care when I read *Being Mortal*, in which Gawande writes,

> We think our job is to ensure health and survival. But really it is larger than that. It is to enable well-being. And well-being is about the reasons one wishes to be alive. Those reasons matter not just at the end of life, or when debility comes, but all along the way. Whenever serious sickness or injury strikes and your body or mind breaks down, the vital questions are the same: What is your understanding of the situation and its potential outcomes? What are your fears and what are your hopes? What are the trade-offs you are willing to make and not willing to make? And what is the course of action that best serves this understanding?[2]

Palliative care—also referred to as supportive care or comfort care—has a clear-cut goal, whether it occurs in conjunction with curative treatments or on its own: to make the patient's life as meaningful as possible, no matter the prognosis, and to provide some relief from the pain and stress associated with a life-threatening illness or injury.

My goal in this book is to help promote the multitude of benefits of receiving palliative care. Even though it is a recognized medical specialty, doctors are highly unlikely to discuss it with their patients. If you find yourself facing a difficult diagnosis, you will have to bring up the subject yourself. As you'll see in the chapters ahead, it is a discussion worth having.

Patients and their families endure a lot as medical professionals attempt to destroy a serious disease. During those curative treatments, palliative care can improve quality of life and help you and your loved ones find meaning in each day together. Regardless of your age or diagnosis, illness should not define you. Palliative care recognizes that essential truth and offers an approach that facilitates living well, even when you're not.

I've written this book to enlighten you about palliative care. I want you to know what it is; how and when to ask for it; why it isn't yet mainstream, even though it is a recognized medical specialty; what the latest medical research says about the benefits of palliative care in serious and terminal illness; and what palliative care can do to benefit not only patients but also their families. You'll even find a checklist to help you prepare for the maelstrom of decisions *before* life starts to spin out of control, as well as how you can find and tap into restorative resources. I also want to debunk the popular misconception that palliative care is only for end-of-life scenarios, such as when a patient is receiving hospice care. Palliative care should be readily discussed with and available to *anyone* who has a serious injury or illness, and that should happen when they are first diagnosed, not in their final days.

This book is also about the importance of hope. We had hope until the moment David died. When you're dealing with an ill loved one, you must never stop working to make the situation better. Hope is what keeps you going. In dire situations, Winston Churchill's words, from a speech he gave in October 1941 during Germany's bombing of England in World War II, say it best: "Never give in. Never give in. Never give in. Never, never, never, never." As soon as you lose hope, everything is lost.

DAVID'S DEATH was ultimately the catalyst that redirected my passion as a health care professional, as a mother, and as a person. He was only one of the millions of Americans in 2000 who faced a life-threatening or terminal illness who did *not* receive palliative care or even know that it existed. That picture has not changed much over the ensuing years. Yet, as medicine offers more and more aggressive treatment options for the seriously ill, palliative care is more important than ever. Concurrent with these advances in medicine is an increase in the number of individuals needing care for serious or life-threatening illnesses; as baby boomers—the largest population group in our history to advance past sixty-five—age, their interaction with health care increases sharply.

I wish we had known about palliative care when David was still with us. However, he lives on as the inspiration for this book and in the work that the Kanarek Family Foundation is doing to take palliative care to a place where it is part of everyone's vocabulary. All of this is part of my ongoing process of healing from the loss of my son. Healing is not forgetting. Healing is not "getting over it." Healing is learning to live life in a way that helps us find meaning. Since David could not contribute more than he did, I can contribute for him. Through this book, I can extend his memory. I think he would be pleased.

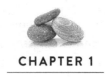

CHAPTER 1

What Is Palliative Care?

We cannot change the outcome, but we can affect the journey.
—ANN RICHARDSON, SOCIAL RESEARCHER AND AUTHOR

An old adage warns, "If you don't ask, the answer is always no."
If you don't know what palliative care is, you aren't going to ask for it, and that means you won't get it. This is a well-established fact, and one that I know from personal experience. By the time you finish reading this chapter, you will know what palliative care is—you may even know more than a lot of health care professionals do about the topic—and you'll know why you should ask for it when you or a loved one encounters a serious illness or injury.

The root of the word *palliative* comes from Latin and means "to cloak." When I first learned of this origin, I pictured someone shivering from exposure to the cold being wrapped in a soft, voluminous blanket. Enveloped by warmth, protection, and a sense of love, the person's shoulders relax as ease and calm begin to return to the body, mind, and spirit. As you'll read in the pages ahead, that image is an apt one to keep in mind while you learn what palliative care is—and what it isn't.

In the United States, palliative care has been a recognized medical subspecialty since 2006. It is not "alternative" medicine, or some kind of voodoo, or an untested fad; it is a board-certified specialty requiring rigorous training, just like cardiology or any other branch of modern medicine. The Center to Advance Palliative Care (CAPC) defines it this way: Palliative care (sometimes referred to in medical circles as PC) is "specialized medical care for people living with a serious illness . . . focused on providing relief from the symptoms and stress of a serious illness. The goal is to improve quality of life for both the patient and the family." That last sentence is key to understanding the purpose of palliative care. Quality of life is the central principle of palliative care. This single-minded dedication springs from the belief that every day of life matters and is a gift that offers the potential for joy. We don't "live" our lives only when we're well; we live life during illness too. Serious illness should not mean an abandonment of one's joy, one's quality of life, one's enjoyment of being alive. This perspective on the human experience is true "health care."

You may be thinking, *This sounds good,* but also wondering, *How is that goal achieved, and what kind of treatment or therapy falls under the auspices of palliative care?* After all, "quality of life" is subjective—what makes life meaningful for me may not be what makes life meaningful for you.

WHOLE-PERSON CARE

One of the key tenets of palliative care is recognizing the unique nature of each individual and acknowledging that "you are not your disease." Palliative care providers start by learning about you the person, as well as about you the patient. Early in your meeting with the team, they'll ask about the things that matter most to you, from the mundane to the sublime—the things that, for you, make each day worth living. These specialists consider your family structure, profession, cultural background, social support system, and spirituality as essential as your medical history. These are the things that make you who you are. They'll also ask you about your fears, pain level, side effects of medical treatments, and all the other variables of your illness that may be degrading your quality of life.

The philosophy behind this approach creates a foundation from which your caregivers can provide you and your family with options that suit your needs now and that can be adapted to those needs as they change, if necessary. This focus on the whole person is where palliative care differs from (and complements) strictly medical or curative care for a serious or life-threatening illness. In conjunction with your doctor's treatment plan, palliative care represents a layer of support to help you enjoy a good quality of life—to the degree to which that is possible—while you undergo treatments that are meant to eradicate or control your disease.

Because palliative care is based on the needs of the individual, the palliative care a woman might receive while going through treatment for breast cancer may be different from the palliative care a man with advanced heart failure receives. But the goal is always the same: to support the best quality of life possible, reduce the physical and mental stress of symptoms, and make interactions with modern medical health care less stressful for the patient and their family.

Who Provides Palliative Care?

Because palliative care focuses on the whole person, it requires an interdisciplinary team of professionals. A basic team includes physicians, nurses, chaplains, and social workers. It may also include pharmacists, behavioral health therapists, physical therapists, and occupational therapists. Generally, urban settings offer more specialties than rural settings do.

Whatever the makeup of the team, everyone works with the patient and their family members to provide a continuum of care that focuses on comfort, support, and quality-of-life issues. Ideally, palliative care begins with the diagnosis of a serious or life-threatening illness so that the person's physical and mental comfort can be maintained and even enhanced during the rigors of curative treatments.

**The World Health Organization's
Definition of Palliative Care**

"Palliative care is an approach that improves the quality of life of patients and their families facing the problem associated with life-threatening illness, through the prevention and relief of suffering by means of early identification and impeccable assessment and treatment of pain and other problems, physical, psychosocial, and spiritual."

World Health Organization, "WHO Definition of Palliative Care," 2013, www.who.int/cancer/palliative/definition/en.

What Types of Palliative Care Exist?

Generalist—also called basic or primary—palliative care is a skill that all clinicians with seriously ill patients should have in order to deliver the fundamentals of palliative care, including managing symptoms, identifying and regularly discussing a patient's treatment goals, and overseeing a transition to hospice. In addition, specialty palliative care, in which palliative care specialists work alongside a patient's primary clinician, even in the earlier stages of illness, has gained more and more traction, particularly since 2013, when the American Board of Medical Specialties granted hospice and palliative medicine formal specialty status. Amid an ever-increasing demand for palliative care providers and the medical field's growing recognition of palliative care's overall value to patients, palliative care specialists serve a useful purpose, especially insofar as some of the skills they provide "are more complex [than those a generalist can offer] and take years of training to learn and apply, such as negotiating a difficult family meeting, addressing veiled existential distress, and managing refractory symptoms."[1]

However, these two branches of palliative care are sometimes at odds. The fact that not enough palliative care specialists exist to meet the needs of every seriously ill patient only underscores the necessity of training generalists in the discipline. But if patients continue to request specialty care regardless of scarcity, "primary care clinicians and other specialists may begin to believe that basic symptom management and psychosocial support are not their responsibility, and care may become further fragmented," say Timothy Quill, MD, and Amy Abernethy, MD.[2] The goal, then, is to seek a coordinated model of care in which the primary medical caregiver is the default provider of palliative care but readily directs patients with more complicated issues to consultations with palliative care specialists. In this arrangement, caregivers on both sides of the fence maximize their skills and their potential to be helpful.

HOW DOES PALLIATIVE CARE IMPROVE QUALITY OF LIFE AND REDUCE THE BURDEN OF SYMPTOMS?

A serious or life-threatening illness or injury elicits universal reactions—fear, distress, confusion—but other responses are specific to the individual, as well as to the nature of the disease and treatments. Let's say your husband has been diagnosed with an aggressive midstage prostate cancer. His urologist and oncologists are recommending a treatment plan of chemotherapy and radiation. Chemotherapy is expected to consist of two sessions per

Palliative Care Goes by Several Names

People use several different terms to talk about palliative care—namely, comfort care, supportive care, and integrative care. I use the term *palliative care* throughout this book. However, if you finish this book and want to do additional reading on the subject—and you should—and you find, for example, an article that uses a different term than *palliative care*, you'll know that it's talking about the same subject we're discussing here.

week for eleven weeks. After that, radiation therapy will be scheduled for five days a week for six consecutive weeks. Both of these treatments can be debilitating, causing nausea, extreme fatigue, diminished appetite, constipation, anxiety, and depression, to name some of the most common reactions. The medical oncologist and radiation oncologist will each be focused on one thing: eradicating the cancer. The unpleasant side effects? Those are too far down the list of urgent priorities for the doctors' attention.

You and your husband want the cancer gone, too. You also want to hold on to some semblance of the life you had as a couple before the diagnosis, to whatever degree that is possible. If, however, neither of you asked for palliative care when you were informed of the curative treatments, it's highly unlikely it will be offered, and the hopes you had to maintain "normalcy" will fade quickly. You will soon find that the side effects of chemotherapy (and, later, radiation) make it nearly impossible for your husband to participate in family life. He is anxious and depressed. As the weeks go by, his personality seems to change; he is becoming short-tempered and lashes out at you almost daily.

Your husband is scared. He's wondering if the treatments will work; if he survives the treatments (which are beginning to feel intolerable), will he be cancer-free or is he facing the beginning of the end? If he does survive, will he ever be able to have sex again? He's worried about his job security; is his company really holding his position until he's well enough to return to work? He's worried about money; is insurance really going to pay for all these bills? He is nauseated much of the time, constipated, not sleeping well, and wondering if he will ever be "himself" again. He doesn't recognize himself when he looks in the mirror.

You're feeling hurt and confused by his behavior toward you, not to mention exhausted by the effort to continue to work, keep the household running, and accompany him to medical appointments. You're also deeply worried about his prognosis and heartbroken to see him suffer.

Meetings with the oncologist feel rushed, and you realize as you are driving your husband home that you both forgot to mention the severe constipation (or other debilitating problem) he has been experiencing.

If you and your husband had asked for palliative care as part of his treatment right from the start, concurrent with his curative care, you and he would be feeling a lot different right now. Of course, you would each still be frightened by the seriousness of the diagnosis and uncertainty of the outcome, but you would be surrounded and supported by a team of professionals whose sole focus is on symptom management—for *both* of you. Their attention to things that your oncologist (or cardiologist, pulmonologist, or any other medical professional providing curative care for a serious or life-threatening illness) is not necessarily thinking about means that you and your husband can still find joy in daily life.

PAIN MANAGEMENT

One of palliative care's primary goals is to manage pain for those who are seriously ill. Although end-of-life care and palliative care both focus on pain and symptom management, palliative care does so along with life-extending disease management. Dame Cicely Saunders—a British nurse, social worker, and, later, physician—who founded modern hospice care in 1967 at London's St. Christopher's Hospice facility—pioneered a concept called total pain, which acknowledges that pain is not just physical but also psychological/emotional, spiritual/existential, and social/interpersonal. As Betty Ferrell, director of the Division of Nursing Research and Education at City of Hope in Duarte, California, explains it, "The experience of pain is an overwhelming, whole-person experience with devastating effects on the experiencing person, the family witness, and the

Palliative Care Clinical Practice Guidelines

In July 2021, the National Comprehensive Cancer Network (NCCN) released a new set of clinical practice guidelines on palliative care in oncology. These recommendations center on palliative care's ability to optimize symptom management and provide patient-centered care that focuses not only on physical, but also on psychosocial and spiritual, needs. They include:

- Patients and their families and caregivers should be told that palliative care is an essential component of comprehensive cancer care.
- All patients with cancer should be repeatedly screened for palliative care needs, beginning with their initial diagnosis and thereafter at intervals as clinically indicated.
- The primary oncology team should initiate palliative care, which is then augmented by collaboration with palliative care experts.
- An interdisciplinary team of palliative care specialists should be available to provide consultation or direct care to patients and/or families as requested or needed.
- All health care professionals should receive education and training to develop palliative care knowledge, skills, and attitudes.
- Institutional quality improvement programs should monitor the quality of palliative care.

M. Dans et al., "NCCN Guidelines Insights: Palliative Care, Version 2.2021," *Journal of the National Comprehensive Cancer Network*, July 28, 2021.

nurse."[3] Chronic pain in any or all areas can cause debilitating changes in someone's personality, lifestyle, function, and ability to socialize. In addition, many patients "consider unrelieved pain as an important factor eroding dignity at the end of life."[4] Palliative care seeks to lessen any symptoms causing suffering and thus to improve patients' ability to function and to maintain their quality of life. Symptoms that palliative care commonly addresses include nausea/vomiting, fatigue, depression and anxiety, insomnia, decreased appetite, constipation, and shortness of breath.

Many different therapeutic options are available for palliative care patients seeking pain management. Depending on the severity of the illness, drug therapy—non-narcotic, narcotic, or adjuvant (steroids, antidepressants, local anesthetics, muscle relaxants, etc.) administered by mouth or under the tongue,

Palliative Care Is *Not* Just for the Dying

Palliative care is an element of health care that is shrouded with misconceptions, the most common being that palliative care is just another term for hospice. One of the most important things you should know about palliative care, therefore, is this: *all hospice is palliative care, but not all palliative care is hospice.*

Palliative care is whole-person care, also often referred to as "comfort care" or "supportive care." It is compassionate, specialized care that is intended to ease pain and improve quality of life. That much of the description of palliative care fits hospice exactly.

Hospice care, however, offers care *only* to those who know their life is ending. There must be a terminal diagnosis with a prognosis of six months or less to live in order for a person to be eligible for hospice care. Hospice *is* for the dying.

Hospice care is usually delivered at home, although it is also available in nursing homes and hospitals; the same is true for palliative care. This, however, is where the similarities end.

Palliative care, on the other hand, is compassionate, supportive comfort care that can begin soon after a person is diagnosed with a serious or life-threatening illness or injury, and it often helps them to endure harsh, curative treatments. Early use of palliative care concurrent with remedial medical care has been shown to not only improve quality of life but also help speed recovery and even extend life. It is appropriate at any age, and at any stage in a serious illness. In other words, palliative care is *not* just for the dying.

intravenously, spinally, or via injection—can be highly effective. For acute, debilitating pain (especially cancer), palliative care experts understand that it is crucial to stay on top of medication administration to maintain therapeutic effectiveness.

However, pain management in palliative care is about much more than medication. Numerous other beneficial therapies can supplement—or, in some cases, even replace—any course of medication and start with focused psychological care: "Short-term psychotherapy, structured support, and cognitive-behavioral therapy can help people develop useful coping skills," says Memorial Sloan Kettering Cancer Center.[5] And cognitive behavioral therapy, which teaches patients to better understand their own responses to and capacity for control over pain, is the most widely used psychological treatment for persistent pain.[6]

Authors Priyanka Singh and Aditi Chaturvedi also cite the following pain-reduction approaches in their article "Complementary and Alternative Medicine in Cancer Pain Management: A Systematic Review" in the *Indian Journal of Palliative Care*:

- **Acupuncture:** Many Western doctors recognize this ancient practice of traditional Chinese medicine as a way to restore the body's energetic balance (or *qi*) and as a complement to conventional medication.

- **Massage:** Manipulating the body's soft tissue can reduce stress and anxiety.

- **Reflexology:** The practitioner applies pressure to specific areas of the body that are believed to correspond to internal organs; the process can relieve stress and decrease pain perception.

- **Yoga:** The *asanas* (poses) in this ancient form of healing movement stimulate muscular development, circulation, and the practitioner's relationship with breathing. Many studies have shown that yoga contributes positively to psychological health and can help to manage symptoms associated with serious illness.

• **Meditation:** Studies show that this mindfulness- and breathing-focused practice can reduce pain and chronic stress for some practitioners.

• **Hypnotherapy:** Hypnosis helps seriously ill patients to address their fear of the unknown, sense of helplessness, and loss of control over their body. It has also been shown to reduce physical pain, fatigue, nausea, and hot flashes.

• **Pet/animal therapy:** Animal-assisted therapy can help relieve patients' physical and emotional suffering.[7] Participating organizations will bring in to hospital units animals meant to boost patients' spirits through companionship, unconditional love, and loyalty.[8]

Many people have a deep-seated fear of pain, especially as they get older, and everyone's pain tolerance is unique. If you are afraid of or have a low tolerance for pain, do not hesitate to share your feelings about that with your palliative care team. They are trained to manage a wide range of responses to pain, but they can't support you unless you vocalize your needs. A lot of people are also concerned about becoming addicted to opioids. This worry is valid, depending on where someone is in the disease process, but especially when you're in the early stages, you certainly don't want to get addicted. You have to explore other options. Your palliative care team is there to spell those out for you so that you can make an informed decision that straddles the line between mitigating your symptoms and keeping you free from chemical dependency for as long as possible.

Whole-Person Care Helps Your Body, Mind, and Spirit (and Your Family's)

It's impossible to anticipate the needs that will arise as you navigate a serious or life-threatening illness or injury. For one thing, you and your family will be reeling from the news of the diagnosis, and the treatments that lie ahead will likely be unfamiliar to you. Palliative care specialists, however, know what you're facing and are familiar with needs you don't even know you'll have. By getting a palliative care team on board as soon after your diagnosis as possible, you'll be putting in place a group of experts devoted to helping you maintain a good quality of life during the arduous journey through curative treatments. While the team will work in partnership with your primary medical doctor, these folks have more time to spend with you, and they know the questions to ask to help you determine what you (and your family) will need to live as well as possible.

Palliative care providers are trained to be skilled communicators, especially during the stress that results from a serious health crisis. No matter how complicated your illness may be or how complex your needs are, they will help you understand what to expect in the days and weeks ahead, and they will ensure that your palliative care plan meets your goals. Pain medication not effective? Trouble sleeping because of anxiety? Overwhelming fatigue? Despondent over missing your gym workouts? Any of these things—and a virtually endless list of others—can be addressed by palliative care.

It is important for the ill person's loved ones to feel supported during this time as well, and the palliative care team can help. Whether it's assistance with insurance forms; getting appointments with the primary medical doctor; ensuring that medical records are being shared across specialties; meeting with a mental health therapist; identifying a support group; finding affordable adult day care; or any number of other nitty-gritty "I need help!" needs that arise, palliative-care givers have answers and resources for you.

WHY DO *YOU* NEED TO KNOW WHAT
PALLIATIVE CARE IS?

If palliative care is a certified medical specialty, recognized by the American Medical Association and offered in fellowship training programs at some of the most prestigious hospitals in the United States; proven to relieve symptoms of serious illness; shown to extend life; and effective at reducing health care costs, why do I want *you* to know what it is? Wouldn't your doctor recommend it to you upon the diagnosis of a serious or life-threatening illness? The short answer to that second question is *no*; your doctor is unlikely to recommend palliative care.

There are a number of reasons why you will most likely not hear about palliative care from your doctor. The most prevalent one is the lack of an accurate understanding of what palliative care is. According to a report published by the American Society of Clinical Oncology (ASCO) in 2018, "Multiple studies indicate that oncologists incorrectly link palliative care with death, dying, hospice, or end-of-life care, and some believe it should be offered only when there are no more cancer-directed therapies available."[9]

Oncologists are not alone in this misunderstanding, and palliative care is certainly not just for those diagnosed with cancer; it is useful for any serious or life-threatening illness, including heart failure, lung disease, and kidney disease, among others.

According to Diane Meier, MD, director emerita of CAPC, most medical specialists are as uninformed about palliative care as the ASCO report shows oncologists are, and for the same reason—they conflate palliative care with hospice. This pervasive misunderstanding among doctors of what palliative care is presents a major impediment for patients. Dr. Meier says, "Physicians are a major barrier to access. They often don't refer [to palliative care], and when patients ask them about it, they say, 'Oh, you don't need that. You're not dying.' "[10]

What Kind of Palliative Care Do You Want?

The kinds of assistance available from a palliative care team are diverse. During your initial meeting with your palliative care case manager, the conversation will include an examination of your medical history, your concerns about the prescribed curative treatments, and your daily habits, professional life, and family life. This discussion will allow the case manager to assemble the providers who will be most helpful to you immediately, and to develop a long-range plan for what may lie ahead. The team will want to know as much about you as possible.

For example, are you someone who suffers from depression? That condition would represent an immediate need for your palliative care team to address. Have you had adverse reactions to narcotic painkillers in the past? This information will be shared with the palliative care physician and pharmacist so that effective analgesics are written into your care plan. Are you concerned about job security as you go through treatment? A meeting with a social worker is needed sooner rather than later. These and many other important matters will be reviewed and addressed. Because the course of an illness and its treatment can mean your needs change over time, the palliative care team will continually check in with you on the many things that can enhance your quality of life. The same attention will be paid to your partner, as that person's role in your journey through illness is invaluable.

No matter what kind of palliative care you need and want, you can be assured the goal of your caregivers is always the same: to help you live well (even when you're not).

That outlook is why Dr. Meier reminds all of us that "you [the patient or family member] have to demand palliative care." She knows from many years as a physician and advocate for palliative care that "if you don't ask, the answer is no."

That same ASCO report cites a public opinion survey that reveals the general US adult population to be equally uninformed, stating, "Few people understand what palliative care is." Interestingly, those surveyed who *had* received early integrated palliative care reported an "appreciation for the quality of life benefits" derived from it.

Those two issues—confusion about palliative care in the medical world and a lack of awareness in the general public—are the reason it's no wonder misinformation surrounds the topic. As I've said—but it can't be overstated—palliative care is *not* another term for hospice. The National Hospice and Palliative Care Organization describes palliative care as an interdisciplinary approach to "patient and family-centered care that optimizes quality of life by anticipating, preventing, and treating suffering."[11] (You will notice there is no mention of dying, death, or end-of-life care in that description.) This goal is achieved with a first step of getting to know the patient. Addressing the person's physical, emotional, psychological, and spiritual needs is of utmost importance in palliative care.

Writing in the *Medical Journal of Australia*, professor Peter Hudson, director of the Centre for Palliative Care in Melbourne and professor at Vrije Universiteit Brussel, and his colleagues echo the idea that "palliative care is too often considered, in the minds of both health care providers and the public, as exclusively about death and dying." The authors describe the following phases of palliative care:

- Early palliative care ("Death is possible"): The main intent is typically curative or life-prolonging (disease-modifying) treatment, but palliative care staff may be involved for symptom management and explaining future palliative care involvement, should this be required.

- Mid-stage palliative care ("Death is probable"): Clinicians would not be surprised if the person died in the foreseeable future (i.e., months ahead). The main focus is therefore a palliative approach, although a number of people will be receiving disease-modifying treatments.

• Late-stage palliative care ("Death is imminent"): The person will likely die soon (i.e., within days or weeks). The focus is therefore entirely end-of-life care.[12]

Although Hudson's insights are not published in a US-based medical journal, the United States would do well to follow the lead of Australia and other countries that are noticeably more progressive in their perspective on and integration of palliative care into their own medical systems.

LIVING WELL MATTERS
(AND SO DOES LIVING LONGER)

If you're thinking, *Comfort is important, but living as long as possible is what matters*, you'll be pleased to know that numerous studies—including one conducted at the renowned Massachusetts General Hospital (MGH) in Boston—indicate that early integration of palliative care for serious or life-threatening illness actually *extends* life.

A study published in a 2017 issue of the *Journal of Clinical Oncology* reported that "early integration of palliative and oncology care in patients with newly diagnosed incurable cancers improves [quality of life], reduces depression symptoms, and enhances coping with prognosis and communication about [end-of-life]-care preferences."[13] Although the authors acknowledge that "further research is needed to define optimal PC delivery models that target the specific needs of different patient populations in the modern era of cancer therapeutics,"[14] their findings clearly highlight the value of integrating palliative care into cancer patients' treatment as early as possible.

According to a 2018 article in *AARP Bulletin* that cited a 2016 *Journal of the American Medical Association* report, palliative care specialists can have an "enormous impact on the quality of your life and your outcomes. When adult patients with blood cancers saw palliative care clinicians at least twice a week during bone marrow transplant procedures, they experienced better symptom control during and after their hospitalization."[15]

It should come as no surprise, then, that as a result of these and other studies, the American Society of Clinical Oncology now recommends that all patients diagnosed with advanced cancer receive palliative care within two months of their diagnosis.

Despite this recommendation to clinicians, you should still plan on asking for palliative care. Also keep in mind that palliative care is appropriate for any serious or life-threatening illness, not just a diagnosis of cancer.

Speaking about the impact of palliative care on longevity, Atul Gawande said in a testimony before the US Senate Special Committee on Aging, "People have priorities in their lives besides just living longer. . . . The overwhelming majority of [the] time, however, we don't ask, whether as clinicians or as family members. When we don't ask, the care and treatments we provide usually fall out of alignment with people's priorities. And the result is suffering. But when we do ask, and work to align our care with their priorities, the results are extraordinary."

He went on to cite a report published in the *Journal of Pain and Symptom Management*, noting,

> We usually don't involve palliative care specialists until the end of life is imminent. There is a common perception among both the medical profession and the public at large that seeking palliative care consultation amounts to "giving up." . . . But the MGH study found that when the [palliative care] specialists were involved early after diagnosis, patients . . . experienced less suffering at the end of their lives, and—here was the kicker—*they lived 25 percent longer*."[16]

Amy Berman, RN: A Nurse's Story

Amy Berman, RN, and senior program officer at the John A. Hartford Foundation in New York City, is a powerful example of the benefits of palliative care. As an advocate for palliative care, Ms. Berman testified before the US Senate Special Committee on Aging. The following is an excerpt from her remarks:

> I'm here because I'm terminally ill. This is the face of somebody who lives with life-limiting illness. . . . Five and a half years ago, I was diagnosed with stage IV cancer—inflammatory breast cancer that spread to my lower spine . . . and this particular kind of cancer has the worst prognosis. . . . The likely course of the disease, 11 to 20 percent [of patients] survive to five years. . . . I'm at five and a half years, and I'm not just here—I'm doing great. I feel well. I work full-time. I get to play and travel and enjoy, walk my puppy, do all of the good things we get to do in life . . . but the reason is because I get the care that most people can't get, the care that isn't yet available. I get access to the workforce that isn't broadly out there. . . .
>
> When I was first diagnosed, I went to two doctors. . . . One doctor wanted to throw everything at the disease, . . . no conversation, never asked me what it is I was hoping to accomplish. . . . He wanted to do the most intense chemotherapy, mastectomy, radiation, and more of the most intense chemotherapy. But unfortunately, there's absolutely nothing that he would have been doing . . . that would have gotten me to a better place, and in fact, it would have gotten me to a worse place.
>
> I went to another oncologist, and [she] explained information in the way in which we talk about [how] care planning should be, talked openly with me about treatment options, and she said, "What is it that you would like to accomplish?" and I said, "Well, I'd kind of like the Niagara Falls trajectory. . . . I want to go 'good, good, good and then drop off the cliff.' Give me more of the good days and try to limit the bad days. That's all that I ask for." . . . Now, that first doctor, who never asked me a question, who suggested what he was going to do to me, not for me, he was going to drop me off the cliff with burdensome treatment, and I was going to go out to the same endpoint. It was the complete opposite of the trajectory that I wanted.

(continued)

It would have been harmful. It would have been costly. I would
have been hospitalized multiple times. . . .

Perhaps the most important aspect of my care, the reason
that I am doing so well despite being seriously ill, is palliative
care. Palliative care is the best friend of the seriously ill. It is an
extra layer of support that goes along with the care provided
by my oncologist. Studies have shown that when palliative care
is added at the beginning of a serious illness . . . people feel
better and live longer.

Ms. Berman not only is enjoying her life but has lived significantly longer than her prognosis predicted. Yes, her cancer is
progressing, but she is able to work, enjoy family and friends, and
pursue her passions. She credits palliative care with the fact that
she is living well, and she intends to do so right up to the end.

Amy Berman, Senate Committee on Aging testimony, June 29, 2016, www
.aging.senate.gov/hearings/the-right-care-at-the-right-time-ensuring
-person-centered-care-for-individuals-with-serious-illness_; "Amy Berman
Tells Senate Committee, 'Palliative Care Is the Best Friend of the Seriously
Ill,'" John A. Hartford Foundation, June 30, 2016, www.johnahartford.org
/blog/view/amy-berman-tells-senate-committee-palliative-care-is-best
-friend-of-the-ser.

A VIEW FROM THE FRONT LINES

As you know from the introduction, my son, David, was never
offered and did not receive palliative care during the extensive
and uncomfortable treatments he underwent for leukemia. We
know he would have benefited from it, as would have every
member of our family.

On one occasion during David's treatment, his dad stepped
in and orchestrated something to address precisely the kind of
quality-of-life issue that palliative care teams handle. It happened following the stem cell transplant. David had been in
the hospital for three weeks when he began expressing more
strongly than ever that he wanted to go home.

That was not a wish his doctors wanted to grant, however, because they were concerned about David's immune system. Prior to receiving the stem cell transplant, David had undergone a round of chemotherapy and radiation therapy to prepare his system for the transplant by essentially eliminating his own immune system. This is standard medical protocol; the intention was to ensure the likelihood that his body would accept—and not attack—the new cells. With a weakened immune system, David was more vulnerable to infection and illness, which was why he had been kept in strict isolation following the transplant and why his doctors wanted him to stay put.

His doctors were pleased with how well David's body responded to the T-cell-depletion stem cell transplant. Three weeks after the procedure, ahead of expectations, David was walking, talking, and acting like himself again and was transferred to a standard room in the pediatric unit. However, one evening shortly after his transfer, he expressed that he was eager to go *home* home, and without further delay. In his usual fashion, he was polite but persistent in the request, and so his dad asked the doctor caring for David if it would be okay. "David would really like to go home, just for tonight. I'll bring him back in the morning," Joe said. David wasn't scheduled for any treatments and was spending most of his time dozing. "Why not let him do that at home?" Joe asked. "It's a forty-minute drive; I'll bring him back immediately if there's any problem," he assured the doctor.

The doctor didn't seem to understand why this visit home meant so much to David. "What is so important about you going home, David? You'll be sleeping most of the time you're there," he said.

"I want to go home, pour myself a tall glass of cold Coke, and watch a movie in the family room with my sister and my dog," David replied.

Sarah, David's sister, was six years younger than David, who was almost fifteen at the time—a tremendous difference in age for an adolescent. Plus, he was a boy and Sarah was a girl, so the details of his wish were disarming to the doctor.

"I've lost this one," the doctor finally said, looking from David to Joe. "Promise me: If you see anything, *anything*, wrong, let me know right away. Bring him right back here."

Joe pulled the car up to the entrance, staff helped get David in the car, and soon they were home. David proceeded to do exactly what he had said he wanted to do, and once he and Sarah were settled comfortably, they did something Joe and I had never seen them do: they started singing their favorite songs together.

When Joe drove David back to the hospital the next morning, David was a changed boy. The amount of energy he had gained by a respite from the hospital setting and one-on-one time with family at *home* gave him a boost that astounded his medical team. Home, after all, is where everyone, including (and especially!) an ill person, wants to be. That single evening had given him back a semblance of normalcy and was a potent medicine for his soul.

As Dr. Atul Gawande shared in his book, *Being Mortal*,

> The terror of sickness . . . is not merely the terror of the losses one is forced to endure but also the terror of the isolation. As people become aware of the finitude of their life, they do not ask for much. They do not seek more riches. They do not seek more power. They ask only to be permitted, insofar as possible, to keep shaping the story of their life in the world—to make choices and sustain connections to others according to their own priorities.[17]

FINAL THOUGHTS

The entire incident of David's brief respite from the hospital setting is an example of what paying attention to quality of life can do for a patient. The focus on each individual's definition of what "quality of life" means is what makes palliative care so powerful and such an important part of a person's journey through serious illness. For our son, it was something as simple as watching a movie in our family room with his sister and his dog. For you, it might be sitting by the ocean or reading your favorite book or having a romantic dinner with your spouse. Whatever your preferences, you should have the option to exercise them, as frequently as you want to, until you reach the end of life. My hope is that this book will give you the confidence to do that.

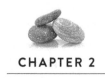

CHAPTER 2

Barriers to Palliative Care

TAKING CARE OF THE PERSON VERSUS FIGHTING THE DISEASE

*The tricky part of illness is that as you go through it, your
values are constantly changing. You try to figure out what
matters to you, and then you keep figuring it out.*

—PAUL KALANITHI (1977–2015), NEUROSURGEON AND AUTHOR
OF THE MEMOIR *WHEN BREATH BECOMES AIR*

When David was diagnosed with leukemia at age ten, we were
grateful that we had access to quality health care and to doctors
whose sole goal was to eradicate his disease. Their focus was
fierce and singular. The gaps in that approach became visible
only over time, when the effects of David's illness and the side
effects of his treatment grew more apparent to us. When he relapsed four years later, in 1999, his diagnosis was even more dire
and his treatments more toxic. Care for his disease clearly began
to occur at the expense of care for his physical, psychological,
social, and spiritual needs.

For example, chemotherapy caused him damage that was
irreversible by the time we caught on to it. Four years into his
treatment, we found out that he had the bones of a ninety-year-
old. His stem cell transplant caused all sorts of other problems
for him. His doctors were so busy with their treatment protocols
that they sometimes seemed to forget that a living patient was
involved. For the first two weeks after his transplant, when he
was in strict isolation, he became so depressed that his entire
personality changed. Yet even then, no one on his medical team

took the time to discuss his distress with him. They were just throwing everything they could think of at the disease, and David got hurt in the process.

The toll that experience took on David and on our family was nearly impossible to endure. Not until some years later, after his death, did we learn it needn't have been that way. If we had known to request that David receive palliative care concurrent with his curative treatments, or if any medical professional had offered us the option, our journey and David's eventual death might have been far less taxing.

Doctors in the United States today feel rushed most of the time. They are expected—by their employer, or by the financial demands of their private practice—to see more patients per day than ever before. In addition, medical school and residency train them to have a single goal: treating their patients' diseases. What they are not taught to incorporate readily into their day-to-day work is whole-person care—which, as we discussed in chapter 1, places a premium on conversing with patients about quality of life when they are grappling with a life-threatening illness or serious injury. As Sunita Puri, medical director of the Palliative Medicine and Supportive Care Service, Keck Hospital and Norris Cancer Center, University of Southern California, observes in her best-selling book, *That Good Night*, medical training taught her that "treating disease was the best way to alleviate suffering" and individual diagnoses became "indistinct."[1] Not until she began a fellowship residency in palliative care did she realize how dehumanizing this perspective was.

When physicians become single-mindedly focused on tackling illness, despite the limits of medical treatment, they will do anything, even at a patient's expense, to eradicate the disease. This one-dimensional approach has numerous negative consequences for the patient, including a decreased quality of life, physical and emotional distress, and a hefty financial burden on both the patient and institutional payors, such as health insurance companies. In short, the burdens that disease-centered care place on a patient can ultimately outweigh the benefits.

The US medical industry has never had a greater need for person- and family-centered care than it does right now. Palliative care focuses on the whole person, and even their family, by recognizing the fundamental human desire for a long and meaningful life. It brings whole-person care to the forefront of a patient's treatment plan—right where it belongs. "Palliative care," says Daniel Johnson, medical director, Supportive Care Solutions, Kaiser Permanente Colorado, "is about delivering comprehensive support centered on what matters most to patients and their families. This whole-person care—whether aimed at relieving physical distress, or providing emotional, spiritual, or practical support—allows individuals to live each day more fully despite serious illness."[2]

Nonetheless, a wide variety of obstacles stand in the way of successful and broad inclusion of palliative care treatment in the United States. The first barrier is a broad lack of public exposure to and knowledge of what palliative care actually is. Several surveys of US adults between 2011 and 2018 revealed that 70 percent of participants were "not at all knowledgeable" about the subject. Of those who had heard the term *palliative care*, the majority of respondents had significant misconceptions of its meaning. Most did not realize that palliative care encompasses not just treatment of symptoms but also bereavement services and spiritual support for patients and their families. More concerningly, many suggested that "palliative care was synonymous with end-of-life care, which was negatively stigmatized to represent death, resulting in avoidance and fear."[3] Importantly, when the survey participants did learn the correct definition of palliative care, 90 percent of them stated that patients, including themselves and their loved ones, should have access to it when appropriate.[4]

The second barrier is that doctors and nurses are not trained in palliative care, which did not even become a defined medical specialty until 2006.[5] The Accreditation Council for Graduate Medical Education currently does not formally require palliative care training within internal medicine, so, writers Mark Hughes and Thomas Smith note, "although primary care physicians may perform palliative care de facto for some of their patients, many . . . may not adequately address certain issues, such as symptom management, spiritual needs, and economic issues."[6] The nationwide lack of programs and guidelines for implementing palliative care in health care settings does a great disservice to any caregiver who interacts regularly with seriously ill patients. Also, as the baby boomer generation continues to age, the number of Americans sixty-five and older is expected to more than double by 2060.[7] As Martha Twaddle, MD, puts it, "We have a tsunami of aging in our world."[8] The higher the concentration of elderly people in the US population, the more terminal-illness cases will exist; thus, the need for palliative care specialists who have all the requisite skills to help this generation achieve a better, more comfortable quality of life as they live out their final years is only going to become more pressing.

Third, the public and medical professionals alike often mistakenly equate palliative care with end-of-life/hospice care, not realizing that "while hospice offers comfort during the last months of life, palliative care can be given at any point in a serious illness—and alongside curative treatment. It is appropriate for any age or diagnosis, from cancer to dementia to heart, kidney, or liver disease," Debra Bradley Ruder explains in a 2015 *Harvard Magazine* article, "An Extra Layer of Care."[9]

Fourth, a doctor may simply not work for an organization that offers palliative care, such as a rural or small hospital. According to CAPC, "Geographic location and regional characteristics influence the availability of palliative care services. People living with a serious illness who reside in the northeastern

United States have access to significantly more hospital palliative care programs than those living in other regions." And while 93.7 percent of hospitals with more than three hundred beds provide palliative care services, only one-third of small hospitals do the same.[10] Even hospitals that do provide palliative care may not make a point of offering it to patients unless they ask for it.

Fifth, overspecialization within today's medical field has yielded an industry of specialists whose knowledge is very deep but also very narrow. In other words, doctors may know a great deal about their own specialty, but that's as far as they can or are willing to go, whereas palliative care, says Twaddle, is an "integrated specialty. It's not another swim lane, so to speak. Medical care is often swim lanes. We're each in our role, we're each in our lane, we do our job. Whereas palliative care is synchronized swimming. The person and family are in the center."[11]

Sixth, some doctors are not comfortable bringing up the subject of death with their patients or fear the patients' and their families' reactions. In addition, many doctors, especially those treating terminal illnesses, perceive death as a failure on their part, so they prefer to continue focusing on medical treatment and to avoid conversations about palliative care altogether.

Finally, medical care teams often suffer from a systemic lack of group communication. Doctors and nurses may document what they see on medical monitors, but they are not willing or equipped to document what patients and their family really want out of treatment for a serious illness or injury. In addition, patients who undergo facilities transitions—such as moving from a hospital to their home, or from a nursing home to hospice—are frequently subjected to a troublesome gap in coordination of care. Each subsequent relocation can cause confusion among the care team, and for the patients themselves, about what the role of each caregiver is. As a result of these pitfalls, patients don't know what questions to ask, what information to seek, or who is their best source of reliable information.

A PATH FORWARD

As we consider all the barriers to widespread availability of palliative care that we must overcome, a number of considerations to prioritize emerge, including the following.

Training

Altering the medical-training landscape is an integral part of overcoming the barriers to widespread availability of palliative care. Everyone who works in the medical field should be educated about what palliative care is and how people can gain access to it, and more physicians, nurses, social workers, chaplains, and other professionals need to specialize in it. "The most promising solution," says Kayla Sheehan, "is to introduce palliative medicine into the medical school curriculum. . . . While improving palliative education at the medical student and resident level may seem an obvious solution . . . , curricular reform is notoriously difficult, and the field of palliative medicine has been unable to compete with other specialties for a four-week block."[12] Efforts to overcome these hurdles are underway. For example, in mid-2021, the University of Maryland announced the addition of a PhD in palliative care to its academic offerings; it will be the first such program in the United States—and, I hope, far from the last. Additionally, in a nod toward the future of medicine, in which artificial intelligence will likely play a more prominent role, the University of Rochester has developed SOPHIE, a virtual patient designed to train doctors to communicate better with their seriously ill human patients about end-of-life matters and to raise awareness of palliative care.[13]

However, palliative care is woefully underrepresented in the vast majority of medical schools. In fact, while conducting research for their 2013 book, *Soul Service: A Hospice Guide to the Emotional and Spiritual Care for the Dying*, Christine Cowgill and Robert Cowgill, MD, "contacted 122 medical schools and 34 of *U.S. News and World Report*'s top 50 nursing schools to obtain information regarding coursework training in the areas of palliative, emotional, and spiritual care to the dying. Only eight of the medical schools and none of the nursing schools contacted had mandatory coursework in those areas of study. Only sixteen of those schools offered elective coursework in those end-of-life care areas."[14]

Medical and nursing schools must expand their curricula to include training, mentorship, and continuing education that centers on emotional and spiritual, not just physical, distress. Not only will giving up-and-coming health care professionals the tools to recognize that their patients are suffering benefit the palliative care population at large, but these professionals themselves may also feel empowered to ponder their own relationships with mortality more deeply. Sunita Puri explains in *That Good Night*, "You either have a deep well of your own suffering—your own intersecting, interlocked circles of loss, grief, anger, fear, sadness, regret—to draw upon, or you have a well of suffering that you have not recognized or are not ready to draw upon. We all have our suffering."[15] The hope is that doctors and nurses who look their suffering right in the eye will, as a result, be less likely to pass on any related issues to their patients and more likely to be successful at person-centered care once they begin their careers.

Empathy

A 2021 Baylor University study, designed to assess whether physician education on how to deliver bad news to seriously ill patients was necessary, indicated that while 91 percent of respondents considered delivering bad news an important skill, only 41 percent believed they were trained to do so.[16] In conversations that center on mortality, doctors must be able to relate to and absorb their patients' distress not in a distant, clinical way, but human to human.

Some helpful resources exist, but sometimes, walking a mile in a patient's shoes is what a physician needs to develop a genuine understanding of that person's struggle.[17] Such is the premise of Atul Gawande's memoir, *Being Mortal*. Gawande was a busy, confident general and endocrine surgeon until his father was diagnosed with cancer and Gawande went to the Midwest to take care of him. Only when he witnessed the limited quality of care that his father was receiving did he develop genuine empathy for his dad's predicament. Since then, Gawande and his colleagues at Brigham and Women's Hospital in Boston have created a "conversation guide" that directs physicians to ask patients important questions about their diagnosis and their mortality, such as "What are your goals for your health situation?" or "What are your biggest fears and worries?" or "What life-extending treatments are you and aren't you willing to undergo?" That approach "doubled the likelihood for documenting patients' preferences for life-sustaining treatment and cut by about half severe to moderate anxiety and depression" among them.[18]

Rana Awdish, MD, medical director of the Pulmonary Hypertension Program of Henry Ford Hospital in Detroit, underwent a similar transformation following a traumatic medical experience of her own. Awdish was a pulmonary and critical care physician—and also seven months pregnant—when a tumor in her liver ruptured. "As a patient," she reflected, "I was privy to failures that I'd been blind to as a clinician. There were disturbing deficits in communication, uncoordinated care, and occasionally an apparently complete absence of empathy. I recognized myself in every failure."[19]

How can we empower more doctors to empathize with their patients, rather than dehumanizing them by reducing them to their diagnosis? In addition to enhanced medical training, a key to achieving this objective is prioritizing time for doctors to really listen. In the traditional model of medical training, Awdish and Leonard Berry explain in the *Harvard Business Review*, "physicians often are taught to maintain a clinical distance and an even temperament. They are warned not to get too close to patients, lest they internalize the suffering and shoulder it themselves." As the medical education field continues to evolve, it needs to instead espouse the view that "actively listening to patients conveys respect for their self-knowledge and builds trust. It allows physicians to assume the role of the trusted intermediary who not only provides relevant medical knowledge but also translates it into options in line with patients' own stated values and priorities. It is only through shared knowledge, transmitted in both directions, that physicians and patients can co-create an authentic, viable care plan."[20] After Awdish's tumor ruptured, her department at Henry Ford formally created a "Culture of Caring," in which "new employees are taught to recognize different forms of suffering: avoidable and unavoidable." The goal is to "find ways to mitigate suffering by responding to the unavoidable kind with empathy and by improving . . . processes and procedures to avoid inflicting the avoidable kind whenever possible."[21] We need more programs like these to help empower physicians, nurses, and other experts to be able to relate to their patients—in short, to make whole-person care their top priority—without having to have firsthand experience with medical trauma.

Standardization of Care

The number of US facilities that offer palliative care is, happily, on the rise. CAPC's 2019 "State-by-State Report Card on Access to Palliative Care in Our Nation's Hospitals" shows "continued linear growth in the number of hospital palliative care teams in the United States."[22] However, standardization of palliative care remains elusive. Diane Meier, CAPC's director emerita, explains, "Physicians do not have to demonstrate core competencies in [palliative care] to be reimbursed. These competencies are akin to those required of a surgeon performing a procedure such as an appendectomy—a procedure that is taught, practiced, and supervised, after which the surgeon's performance is assessed for quality and safety before he or she is allowed to perform it independently."[23] Would you want your appendix removed by a doctor who wasn't even qualified to do the procedure? Certainly not—so why should any patient seeking palliative care not be guaranteed universally high-quality treatment in that area when they need it most? That's a rhetorical question, but until standardized palliative care becomes the norm, rather than the exception, many patients will continue to fall victim to such troubling factors as "variation in quality and access . . . , confusion over whether and how best to measure and report quality of care for seriously medically ill people, a lack of confidence among the public that doctors and nurses have the necessary clinical competencies, and the continuation of well-documented overuse of low-value and burdensome medical interventions among patients who cannot benefit from them."[24]

The good news is that robust efforts to enforce quality control among hospitals, home-based organizations, and individual providers of palliative care are underway. For one, the National Consensus Project for Quality Palliative Care has released *Clinical Practice Guidelines for Quality Palliative Care,* 4th edition, a "blueprint for excellence by establishing a comprehensive foundation for gold-standard palliative care for all people living with serious illness, regardless of their diagnosis, prognosis, age or setting." More than ninety US medical organizations endorse this resource.[25] And numerous other organizations are spearheading palliative care certification and accreditation programs, designed to reduce variations in palliative care protocols; promote interdisciplinary communication; and cater to patients' physical, intellectual, emotional, social, and spiritual needs. These programs include Joint Commission palliative care certification; Community Health Accreditation Partner palliative care certification; Accreditation Commission for Health Care's palliative care distinction; and various certification programs for specific practitioners, such as physicians, nurses, social workers, and chaplains. The more public awareness of these initiatives we can generate, the more their mission is likely to become standard practice in the health care system. Hospitals and other medical organizations respond to pressure from the public. If the public is demanding something that they're not providing, those patients will look elsewhere. Any patient who is currently seeking palliative care and doesn't know where to begin will find the most comprehensive information on CAPC's website, GetPalliativeCare.org.

Awareness of Financial Benefits

Health care costs for individuals and institutions increase each year, and the United States has long spent the most money per capita on health care. People living with serious illness have to rely frequently on the system for care, and they are suffering financially for it. A 2018 survey of the country's most gravely ill people, conducted by the *New York Times*, the Commonwealth Fund, and the Harvard T. H. Chan School of Public Health, revealed that 36 percent of people *with* health insurance had spent all or most of their savings on health care costs, and 21 percent could not pay for necessities like food, heat, and housing.[26]

A popular misconception within the US medical field is that palliative care will only increase these already untenable costs, when in fact the opposite is true. The seventy-plus countries in the world that practice socialized medicine already know this, but the United States is lagging far behind. In an attempt to change our flawed financial model, abundant studies are comparing expenditures for patients who do have palliative care as part of their treatment plan with those who do not, and the contrast is startling.

First, palliative care drastically lowers hospital readmission rates for patients, among other benefits, CAPC explains.

"Reducing readmissions is currently part of a national strategy to reduce health care costs, the main target being 30-day readmission rates. Palliative care programs help to reduce readmissions by 50%."[27] Patients receiving home-based palliative care simply do not need to go to the hospital, even shortly before their death, as much as their counterparts do, because the quality of life they are enjoying at home gives them the sense of safety and comfort they need during their final months. And even when end-of-life palliative care patients are hospitalized, their costs for an inpatient visit are significantly lower: $1,137, versus $5,946 for patients not receiving palliative care.[28] Overall, by 2040, palliative care could reduce health care costs in the United States by a staggering $103 billion, or $4,000 average per patient.[29] For patients who are already under great emotional and physical duress, not to mention confused by the often maddening process of navigating the US health care system, that cost savings has a value that extends far beyond its monetary worth.

Coordinated Communication and Care

When someone today has a significant illness, a doctor is not the only person that patient communicates with. They also have contact with nurses, therapists, social workers, chaplains, and other professionals. However, rather than working as a cohesive team, these experts far too often fail to communicate with one another and, worse, with their patients themselves. We need to create a culture in the US medical system that ensures that palliative care and advance care planning are always an early part of any conversation about a patient's treatment plan—or, better yet, part of a regular conversation that anyone over age fifty, including people who are not currently ill, has with their medical team. If the doctor doesn't bring it up, the nurse should; if the nurse doesn't bring it up, the social worker should, and so on. And in an ideal future, every care team will include at least one palliative care specialist who can guide the others in coordinating treatment and communication for the greatest benefit to the patient.

This is one of the reasons Joe and I funded the integration of pediatric nurse practitioners into an educational program called Comskil, whose goal was to teach clinicians advanced communication skills for interacting with cancer patients and their families, at Memorial Sloan Kettering Cancer Center from 2011 to 2016. Prior to that period, Comskil was dedicated to educating fellows, surgeons, and physicians only; nurses were not being utilized, even though they were the ones whom the patients sought out when they needed more information on difficult subjects. Our support ushered in the first cohort of nurses learning these core skills. VitalTalk, established in 2005 by three seasoned academic doctors with extensive National Institutes of Health research funding, is another excellent program primarily for clinicians who need to learn how to communicate effectively and sensitively in difficult conversations.[30] The organization's mission statement explains,

> We know and believe that effective, empathic, and honest conversations between a clinician, patient, and their family are the cornerstones of patient-centered care. Just as no doctor is born knowing how to handle a scalpel, the same is true for communicating effectively with patients. But, despite best efforts, too few clinicians are trained on or get to practice critical patient conversations. . . . Our approach draws on a unique educational philosophy built on empirical research of proven strategies to combat communication pitfalls.[31]

When the time comes for a patient to transition from, for example, an in-patient hospital setting to a skilled-nursing facility and then home, Twaddle emphasizes the importance of staff cooperation to ensure a "warm handoff." She says, "We know that people with serious illness . . . are very vulnerable when they move . . . [and] that at those points of transition, care plans can deteriorate." Twaddle recommends that a skilled palliative care provider from the patient's previous facility not only give staff at the next facility clinical information about the patient but also talk "about who they are and what [the caregiver has] learned about them and their family"—in other words, the emotional and spiritual nuances of a person.[32] A good-faith gesture like this can make a world of difference in the patient's sense of ease and adaptation to their new environment.

Unfortunately, as long as the current model of care precludes this kind of coordinated effort and communication across the board, medical teams are unlikely to bring up the subject of palliative care with their patients, so it is up to the patient to ask for it. There's a phrase in the Talmud that essentially says, "If I'm not for myself, then who is?" As I will underscore again and again, you have to fight for yourself. That is why I am writing this book—to educate the public about how and when to advocate for themselves and to request—no, to *demand*—palliative care as soon as they are diagnosed with a serious illness, not when they are reaching the end of life. Yes, we are all going to die someday, so that understanding should be implicit in any conversation with a person with a life-threatening condition. And yes, modern medicine can keep people alive for an extended period of time. Yet most of the patients currently on ventilators in an ICU somewhere are not likely to say that is how or where they want to spend their last days. Regardless of how much time someone has left, they deserve a conversation that centers not on death but on how they want to *live*. Too often, no one has asked them that question.

If you have been diagnosed with a serious illness, you owe it to yourself to tell your doctor, your nurses, your therapist, your chaplain, and anyone else on your care team what your definition of "quality of life" is, and to ask them what kind of support system they can offer you to help you achieve it. We'll discuss this topic further in chapter 4: "How to Get the Care You Want."

FINAL THOUGHTS

For those of us who have been diagnosed with a serious illness, treatment of our condition is mostly up to our physicians and, in many cases, is out of our hands. We have few or no choices left. But how we live in the time we have remaining *is* still up to us. Palliative care is about how we can best make that choice and help other people to support us in doing so. Or, as Sunita Puri puts it, "Palliative medicine is bridging articulation and action. It means helping people to really specify what they mean when they use certain words, what they mean when they articulate certain goals, and bridging them from where they are now to a place closer to those goals. But it also means being honest when we are coming up against a limit."[33] If we are to be a culture of caring, not just curing, we must do everything we can to urge our medical institutions and our caregivers to be more compassionate, more inquisitive, more attuned to our individual needs and wishes—once again, more committed to treating a whole person, not merely their disease. We have only one life to live, and this is our chance to make it as meaningful as possible in whatever time we have left. What could be more important than that?

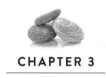

CHAPTER 3

How We Want to Die

PALLIATIVE CARE'S BENEFITS FOR PATIENTS
AND THEIR LOVED ONES

Life is not separate from death. It only looks that way.
—BLACKFOOT INDIAN PROVERB

"I certainly—if I can help it—don't want to die in any institution. I want to be at home."

"I don't want my final days to be characterized by the presence of any doctor or medical personnel, except perhaps a hospice nurse."

"I would want to be at home, if I can, and to have the people I care about with me."

"I definitely would want my symptoms controlled, and I want my doctor to let me know when it's time to go fishing."

"It's going to be somewhere other than the hospital."

"In my bedroom, making love to my spouse."

"I've already told my children I will not die in a hospital; that's just verboten."

Such are the responses of doctors when asked how *they* would like to die, sparked by a nationwide discussion of the 2011 essay "How Doctors Die," by Ken Murray, MD.[1] In that piece, Murray describes how, "for all the time they spend fending off the deaths of others, [doctors] tend to be fairly serene when faced with death themselves. They know exactly what is going to happen, they know the choices, and they generally have access to any sort of medical care they could want. But they go gently."

It's no surprise, then, that doctors are more likely to die at home with less aggressive care. One study, led by Harvard Medical School researchers, confirms that physicians are statistically less likely than the general population not only to die in a hospital but to have surgery in the last six months of life or be admitted to the ICU.[2]

According to another study, published by Stanford University School of Medicine, most physicians would opt for a "no-code" (also known as DNR, for "do not resuscitate") directive for themselves if they were terminally ill. And the kind of care they want when they have a serious or terminal diagnosis (or when the body is simply succumbing to the ravages of advanced age) is palliative care at home. Yet they pursue aggressive, debilitating treatments for their patients facing the same diagnosis, and less than 10 percent of doctors will ever have a conversation with their patients about death.

Murray makes a fair point, that it's "easy to find fault with both doctors and patients in such stories, but in many ways all the parties are simply victims of a larger system that encourages excessive treatment."[3] Nevertheless, the gap between how doctors themselves want to be treated and how they treat their patients can feel vast and unbridgeable. How do most people who are *not* doctors die, or spend their final months and weeks after a terminal diagnosis? Studies show that while most Americans state a preference to die at home without life-prolonging interventions, 80 percent do not have that opportunity. Most Americans (60 percent) die in hospitals, surrounded by strangers in a loud environment and often hooked up to life support; another 20 percent die in nursing homes; and only 20 percent die at home.[4]

Palliative care delivered at home should be the norm for anyone who has a life-threatening condition. Palliative care's goal of living a good life, whether it is used in conjunction with curative care or instead of it, gives us the dignity and opportunity to make whatever time we have more meaningful. This chapter will illuminate the most significant ways in which palliative care can help patients and their family members alike, as well as the importance of planning in advance for end-of-life scenarios.

THE FACTS

The Center to Advance Palliative Care (CAPC) has some helpful statistics on the intersection of illness and palliative care in the United States, including the following:

- "Approximately 90 million Americans are living with serious illness, and this number is expected to more than double over the next 25 years with the aging of the baby boomers."

- "Approximately 6,000,000 people in the United States could benefit from palliative care."

- Patients who benefit most from palliative care are those suffering from "heart disease, cancer, stroke, diabetes, renal disease, Parkinson's and Alzheimer's disease."

- "Palliative care is appropriate at any age and at any stage in a serious illness, and it can be provided together with curative treatment."[5]

Note that the list above specifies that palliative care applies to a *wide range of diseases, ages, and stages of illness*. People have gotten the idea that palliative care is for cancer patients, and PC *has* traditionally been used in cancer settings, but all the research is showing that we're going to have to integrate it across all branches of medicine. Since I began advocating for palliative care awareness, all kinds of physicians working outside the field of oncology—especially cardiologists, neurologists, and

transplant doctors—have contacted me to express their gratitude for anything people can do to acknowledge the need for
palliative care's diffusion into broader medicine, as they don't
know how to make that happen themselves within their area of
specialization.

The reason palliative care is thought of as being utilized
mostly for cancer patients is that cancer is not a disease that
kills people overnight. Many times, the period from diagnosis
to death is months, if not years. However, this same trajectory
occurs in numerous other health circumstances as well. For
example, people can be ill for years with kidney problems, heart
problems, and lung problems, due to decades of organ abuse.
People also suffer for long periods from Parkinson's disease,
Alzheimer's disease, multiple sclerosis, traumatic brain injuries,
childhood cancer, or young-adult cancer. For all these patients,
palliative care has tangible benefits, chiefly the following:

- regular access to specialists trained to deal with complex
  pain and symptoms, as well as in the art of communication about serious illness

- help with a wide range of issues, including pain, depression, anxiety, fatigue, shortness of breath, constipation,
  nausea, loss of appetite, and difficulty sleeping

- increased strength to carry on with daily life

- higher tolerance for medical treatments

- more control over one's care by improving one's understanding of treatment options and matching their goals
  to those options

- support for family caregivers, and practical wisdom[6]

The advantages are undeniable, but we need to push for more
in-depth research on how palliative care affects quality of life

specifically for patients who do *not* have cancer. The preliminary results are somewhat sparse but promising. When it comes to Parkinson's disease and related disorders (PDRD), for instance, while few studies are available to quantify palliative care's effectiveness as an intervention, one clinical trial, held between 2015 and 2017, concluded that "the integration of PC into PDRD care holds the potential to improve outcomes, particularly for persons who are underserved by current models of care. . . . A need exists to optimize the intervention, particularly for caregivers, and to develop models appropriate for implementation in non-academic settings and among diverse populations."[7] The same is true for traumatic brain injury (TBI); one group of experts says,

> Recent studies have [emphasized] the growing needs for palliative care services among patients with neurologic diseases. . . . Interventions provided through palliative care services can play a crucial role in enhancing TBI patients' and caregivers' quality of life, decision-making, and emotional distress. Furthermore, the expected increase in TBI rates over the next few years, with the concomitant growth of their cost of care, requires implementing different strategies to help in reducing the economic burden associated with this condition. It is possible that the early integration of palliative care in the care of these patients could aid in lowering their health care costs and improving outcomes.[8]

Another study found that patients suffering from dementia or organ failure had a very different experience with palliative care than cancer patients did—because palliative care began earlier for the latter than for the former and because more patients with terminal noncancer illnesses died in the hospital, even when palliative care was initiated at home for them.[9] No matter what a patient's condition, the timeline for care and planning should not differ significantly across the medical field.

Milestones in the areas of end-of-life and preventive care are also occurring. First, the Affordable Care Act (ACA) was passed in 2010, during Barack Obama's presidency, and significantly expanded access to high-quality end-of-life care for seriously ill Americans. The increased availability of such care arose from two alarming circumstances: first, almost 715,000 people died in US hospitals each year, rather than at home, and second, fewer than half of people on Medicare took advantage of hospice services, even though hospice helps patients to have a better quality of life and supports their loved ones in the grieving process. The ACA seeks to remedy those statistics, because "integrating specialty palliative care with standard oncology care in adults leads to significant improvements in quality of life and care without a survival decrement," and because "the improved outcomes associated with early, concurrent palliative care likely lead to reduced health care spending and utilization in both inpatient and outpatient settings."[10] To address the financial part of that equation specifically, the Obama White House also passed Title IV: Prevention of Chronic Disease and Improving Public Health, which increased prevention and wellness coverage for Medicare beneficiaries.

At the Centers for Disease Control and Prevention, officials have made similar moves in the preventive-care arena by founding a Division for Heart Disease and Stroke Prevention. This initiative encourages self-management of health by supporting "state, local, tribal, and territorial heart disease and stroke prevention programs that help millions of Americans control their high blood pressure and reduce other risk factors for heart disease and stroke"—namely, high blood pressure, high LDL cholesterol, cigarette smoking, poor nutrition, lack of physical activity, type 2 diabetes, and obesity—especially among groups affected by health disparities based on geographic, ethnic, socioeconomic, and other factors.[11]

In 2017, the US Senate Committee on Finance passed the CHRONIC Care Act, granting senior citizens with kidney disease access to telehealth at home for the first time. Then, in 2020, the CARES Act allowed Medicare providers to offer all seniors telehealth services, regardless of geographic location, as well as allowing Federally Qualified Health Centers to receive payments for telehealth from Medicare. These two acts represent a major step toward enabling more seriously ill Americans to get what most of them want, which is information and treatment in the comfort of their own homes. Other federal organizations promoting positive change in chronic disease include the Partnership to Fight Chronic Disease, the Agency on Aging, the National Institutes of Health, the National Council on Aging, and the Patient-Centered Outcomes Research Institute.

HIGH NEEDS, HIGH COSTS

The United States is home to an alarming number of high-need patients. More than twelve million Americans are dealing with three or more chronic health conditions and are functionally limited in their ability to care for themselves; a 2016 study found that 5 percent of the US population, ages eighteen and up, falls into this category.[12]

Three key variables identify the high-need population:

1. Diagnosis
   - cancer
   - advanced liver disease
   - chronic obstructive pulmonary disease with use of oxygen
   - heart failure
   - renal failure
   - advanced dementia
   - diabetes with complications
   - ALS (Lou Gehrig's disease)

2. Functional impairment
   - limitations in activities of daily living: eating, bathing, dressing, toileting, transferring, and walking
   - significant memory loss
   - use of durable medical equipment—walkers, beds, home oxygen, and so forth
3. High utilization
   - more hospital admissions/readmissions; longer hospital stays
   - more emergency department visits
   - more polypharmacy (the simultaneous use of multiple drugs to treat a medical condition)
   - more skilled-nursing-facility/rehab stays
   - more multiple home-care episodes

Currently, a staggering 71 percent of US total health care spending is directed toward Americans with more than one chronic condition—as of 2018, one in four US adults had two or more chronic conditions and more than half of older adults had three or more, though these people are not considered high-need, as they can still function fairly well—and the high-need patients are costing the health care system even more money than these adults with multiple chronic conditions only.[13] Annual health care expenditures among the high-need population are nearly three times higher, and their out-of-pocket expenses are more than one-third higher, than those of their counterparts; they're using hospitals more than twice as much; and they visit doctors and use home health care more often.[14] As the Partnership to Fight Chronic Disease put it in 2016, "The escalating burden of chronic conditions is unsustainable."[15] Thus, as the health care industry assesses how to more broadly integrate palliative care into hospitals, homes, and other facilities, it must devote special consideration to this particular demographic. These are the people who desperately need both aggressive symptom management *and* the benefits of the team-based, interdisciplinary approach that palliative care embraces—*well before* the last six months or so of a person's life, or before a patient enters hospice. Of course, people preferably take responsibility for their health for their entire life span so that they don't find themselves grappling with multiple chronic conditions in the first place, but when they don't have that option anymore, the earlier palliative care is integrated, the easier it will make their lives.

THE CONSEQUENCES OF SILENCE

Unfortunately, as we've discussed, one of the main dilemmas plaguing the health care industry today is that many people don't even know that palliative care is something they should want, because of the misconceptions surrounding it (that it's only for hospice or end-of-life patients), because of lack of awareness about it (see chapter 2), or because of a lack of willingness—on the part of patients and doctors alike—to talk about it. The truth is, a lot of patients simply aren't willing to verbally acknowledge the subject of their own mortality. In a 2019 survey, geriatrician Nancy Schoenborn asked a group of 878 people ages sixty-five and older how they would feel discussing their life span with their doctors if they were hypothetically going to die earlier than their peers because of serious health issues. The patient in this scenario would have multiple chronic health conditions, but those would be well managed by medical intervention, and thus the time they have left to live would not be top of mind. Essentially, this is a patient like the ones I encountered when I was a diabetes educator, who think, *My kidneys are failing, but I'm on dialysis, so I'm going to live to be in my eighties or nineties*, without any understanding that this disease can kill them.

Of the respondents to Schoenborn's survey, 59 percent said they would not like to talk with their doctor about their expected life span under those circumstances; moreover, 60 percent of that segment wouldn't want their doctor even to ask for permission to discuss the topic, and 88 percent would not want the doctor discussing their life expectancy with their families.[16] The fact that only about one in ten doctors have conversations with their patients about death and the fact that Medicare does not pay doctors to have end-of-life planning discussions with patients only exacerbate the situation.[17]

What happens if patients and their doctors don't have this crucial talk, and if they aren't proactive about advance care planning when they're still reasonably sound of body and mind, is that they're eventually thrown into a situation where their condition is dire and drastic measures are going to have to be decided upon, and that's when people panic. For example, I went to my hairstylist one day. She knew about my nursing experience, and she knew I was writing this book, and she said, "I need your advice." Her best friend's mother, who was in her early eighties, had had diabetes for years and had recently entered kidney failure. After a difficult hospitalization, in which she developed a leg ulcer and had to have her leg amputated, she was finally discharged home. When a nurse arrived to follow up, she was shocked to discover that the patient's discharge plan included no indication of the amputation. Not only did the woman need a dressing change for her wound, but she had developed a bed sore on her sacral area. She was in severe pain and beginning to dream about reuniting with family members—frequently a sign that death is near.

When my hairstylist asked me, "How can I help?" I said, "I have to be honest—it doesn't sound like this woman has very long to live. This is not going to get better. It's only going to get worse. I'd recommend that she talk immediately with her doctor about hospice care, as well as about how she wants to live the remainder of her life. And if the doctor is not comfortable, I have a friend who's a palliative care physician who can talk to the family and guide them, along with the general practitioner, about the outcomes for this woman."

This is what we are up against right now. Until palliative care is mainstream, the loved ones of patients are going to find themselves in this kind of dilemma with unique-needs patients, wondering how to help and not even knowing where to begin. Where people should begin is by summoning the courage to have a conversation with their health care providers *as early as possible* about quality of life as they age. Ideally, this dialogue would be a routine part of an annual physical exam, when the patient is still healthy; however, regardless of setting, it's fundamentally about stating preferences, such as "I do not want to be resuscitated in such-and-such circumstance," "I need help writing an advance directive," or "I want palliative care to be part of my treatment plan." (We'll delve more deeply into how to have this discussion in chapter 6, "Putting It All Together.") Katie Butler, author of *Knocking on Heaven's Door: The Path to a Better Way of Death* and *The Art of Dying Well: A Practical Guide to a Good End of Life*, says,

> The communication between doctors and patients around end-of-life questions is absolutely terrible. It's almost as if we need a foreign-language phrase book. For instance, if the doctor says, "I want to talk to you about your goals of care," the patient might well not understand that the doctor is probably saying, "The time you have ahead of you appears to be limited, and, given that, how do you want to spend your time? Do you want to take a trip, or see a child graduate? Can medicine help you achieve this? And, if not, what are some achievable goals?"[18]

In a perfect world, the medical field will reach a point where no such "phrase book" is necessary because patients and doctors understand each other perfectly, and because doctors are automatically initiating these exchanges with their patients early on. Atul Gawande believes that every patient should be asked five questions about their priorities as they near the end of life. For example, he tells the story of a woman who had been undergoing treatment for incurable cancer for two years. By the time her doctors asked her what she really wanted out of the life she had remaining, she said she wanted to take her grandchildren to Disney World. But she never had the chance to do so, because no one asked her that question until it was too late. The woman died just a few days after she had this conversation with her doctor.[19]

To reduce the occurrence of such avoidable tragedies, Gawande began training physicians to ask their patients a series of five questions:

1. What is your understanding of where you are and of your illness?

2. What are your fears or worries about the future?

3. What are your goals and priorities?

4. What outcomes are unacceptable to you? What are you willing to sacrifice and not?

5. What would a good day look like?

Gawande says, "This is not just a conversation doctors have; any family can have it, too. It's not just about the last weeks of life, it's about the last decade. . . . [This is] the conversation that has to become normal in our country and in the world."[20]

Until that day comes, though—until all doctors are as comfortable as Gawande's trainees at bringing up tough topics—the onus is on patients to be proactive about asking questions. If the woman with kidney failure whom I described above had spoken with her doctors much earlier in her illness, she and her care team would have been more ready for the time when her condition became more acute. And if she had employed at least some palliative care measures throughout her illness, rather than just at the end, she might have had a better result. Keep in mind that the dying process doesn't happen overnight. As Yale University surgeon and ethicist Sherwin Nuland wrote in his seminal book, *How We Die*, the human body has many systems—cardiovascular, renal, pulmonary, neurological—and they all break down at different times. A chronic illness like diabetes, which this woman had, is different from a terminal illness like cancer. When you're diagnosed with cancer, you're just thrown into it, right off the deep end. With chronic illnesses, you theoretically have time to prepare—yet this woman had no such luck, because no one prompted her to reflect on and then clearly vocalize her wishes.

ADVANCE CARE PLANNING IS FOR EVERYONE

It's also important to note that talks about advance care planning and palliative care don't need to occur solely with older patients, although that has been the trend. A group of researchers studying geriatric palliative care submit that while "researchers and clinicians alike [must] recognize the implications of missed opportunities to engage older patients in PC," health care providers must also realize that "patients of all ages would be better served by having GOC [goals-of-care] discussions earlier on in the illness trajectory, as accurately anticipating patient preferences is not always straightforward."[21] For children, adolescents, and young adults with complex chronic conditions and terminal illnesses, as well as their parents, advance care planning is a vital component of optimal care. In a survey of 114 bereaved parents with children in this category, all parents reported that advance care planning was important, and 70 percent stated that such conversations should occur early after diagnosis. Sixty-five percent of the respondents said that advance care planning had helped them to feel prepared for their child's last days of life and to rate their child's end-of-life quality as good to excellent."[22]

The aggressive treatment approach that many doctors are trained to take by default in an attempt to preserve, not destroy, life makes advance care planning especially urgent for patients' families. Ken Murray describes an all-too-real scenario in which

> someone has lost consciousness and been admitted to an emergency room. As is so often the case, no one has made a plan for this situation, and shocked and scared family members find themselves caught up in a maze of choices. They're overwhelmed. When doctors ask if they want "everything" done, they answer yes. Then the nightmare begins. Sometimes, a family really means "do everything," but often they just mean "do everything that's reasonable." The problem is that they may not know what's reasonable, nor, in their confusion and sorrow, will they ask about it or hear what a physician may be telling them. For their part, doctors told to do "everything" will do it, whether it is reasonable or not.[23]

Well before they find themselves in this kind of grim situation, patients and their loved ones need to define what "reasonable" means for them personally, and to communicate those parameters to their health care providers. The amount of intervention a family wants means having a wide-ranging conversation about death—no matter how uncomfortable it is.

That was not our experience when David was diagnosed with leukemia. Instead, the first doctor who took care of him said simply, "I can arrest this disease." There was very little talk along the lines of "The percentage of children who survive this form of cancer is high, but there's a reasonable chance this is not going to work out and David is going to die." I was with David in the doctor's office in Connecticut, and Joe was on a trip in California, so she probably said this partly so Joe wouldn't panic and fly home. He describes doing just that, though; "I flew home that night and was in a cold sweat the whole way. I knew cancer kills people," Joe recalls.

At first, Joe and I didn't want to have a discussion about the end of David's life; we were focused solely on holding on to hope. We had a few talks about planning for contingencies, but they were short and we mostly pushed any bad thoughts out of our minds. In retrospect, though, when David relapsed, it would have been nice to have had a handout, of sorts—really, a book like this—to help us clarify what our options were.

We didn't receive confirmation that David was going to die until his last two weeks of life. He had just moved from Memorial Sloan Kettering Cancer Center to New York-Presbyterian Hospital, and all the doctors to whom we had entrusted his care for the past six months at MSK practically stopped communicating with us. They were just across the street, but it felt like they already knew that he was going to die and they didn't want to face us—or their own failure to cure him. His new care team didn't know us at all, and we didn't know them.

David was very ill and coughing up blood. One morning at six o'clock, when I was at home and Joe was alone with David in his room, a doctor whom Joe had never laid eyes on before came in and said, "I want to talk to you." Joe went into a conference room with him, and without any warning he blurted out, "Your son is going to die."

Before Joe could even get his mind around what he had just heard, the doctor asked cursorily, "Are you okay?"

In a departure from his usually easygoing personality, Joe raised his voice and said, "No, I'm not okay! You're telling me out of the blue that my son is going to die, and then you're asking me if I'm going to be okay?"

After Joe said his piece, the doctor neither hurried to respond nor showed any sign of real emotion, for that matter. Joe got up and left the room, thinking, *Maybe this man is a "good doctor," but what a miserable human being. He delivered a terrible message to me, without any attempt to even fake empathy. "Are you okay?" Really? Now, that's a winner!* There were so many other, more humane ways this doctor could have delivered this fatal blow, such as by saying, "I'm sorry, but it looks like there is nothing more we can do to save your son." This encounter was a glaring example of the mechanical approach most members of a so-called "healing profession" employ, rather than showing their humanity. Most people would have shown more concern to someone with a paper cut on their finger.

Things got even worse from there. David developed a lethal fungal infection in his lungs, and his doctors said they had to intubate him and send him into a medically induced coma. They told Joe and me that we should tell David he was going to die, right before they put the tube down his throat. I said, "Are you kidding me?" What was David going to do with that knowledge? For him, being intubated wasn't a tragedy—it was simply going to make him feel better because he'd be able to breathe again. So if we had told him right before he was put under that this was his last conscious moment on Earth, what would that have accomplished? Where was the logic in that?

Up until the moment of his death, we were hopeful that something miraculous would happen, but the day before he died, a senior resident talked to me for a long time. I said to him, "I need you to be honest with me. What are the chances that David is going to be able to recover from what he is going through and lead a normal life?"

The resident said, "On top of the stem cell transplant, your son is going to need a double lung transplant, and he's probably going to need a kidney transplant." And he'd probably be in a wheelchair because his bones were so brittle. That was when I realized that David, even if he survived, would be at the mercy of health care for the rest of his life. In short, his life would be awful.

That was when Joe and I decided that we were going to establish parameters in David's treatment plan, and that if his heart were to stop, we'd have a do-not-resuscitate order in place and we'd let him go. That was what we did, and our beloved son died very peacefully as a result.

My point in sharing this story is to illustrate that at critical moments in a patient's life—such as during Joe's interaction with the doctor in the conference room, and during my exchange with the resident—a doctor who knows how to present such difficult information is invaluable, and also quite rare. I made David's doctor's job easier because I posed the most important question to him myself—I had the courage to ask what my son's quality of life would be. He didn't bring it up on his own. I suspect it will take at least another several years, as of 2023, for doctors to be the ones to ask patients and their families the right questions without prompting, but we need to start thinking today about what those questions are.

THE DOCTOR-PATIENT DIVIDE

Another essential question to keep asking is why the end-of-life approach doctors would choose for themselves differs so radically from the way they treat their terminally ill patients. We know from the Stanford study cited at the beginning of this chapter that nearly 90 percent of physicians would not want to be treated aggressively, endure prolonged hospitalization, or be resuscitated if they were terminally ill. Yet the vast majority of the time, they resort to excessive lifesaving measures for patients with a similar prognosis, even when those patients would not choose to endure such an experience.

The answer to this question is multipronged. First, and most fundamentally, doctors are trained to prolong life, not to end it. Deciding not to resuscitate a dying patient—indeed, even having a conversation about mortality with a patient—flies in the face of their education. As a result, doctors end up putting on blinders to patients' individual wishes about what they're willing to tolerate in end-of-life scenarios.

Second, money plays a part, in a few different ways. US health insurance centers on a fee-for-service model that compensates doctors for quantity, not quality, of treatment. Higher-volume physicians get paid more than those who spend extra time with their patients. The reality is that many doctors are going to choose money over in-depth, personal interactions. Patient litigation is another concern; if health care providers are worried about being sued for patient negligence or medical malpractice, they're going to err on the side of excess when it comes to treatment. Finally, the Stanford study, which focused on doctors and lawyers, highlighted the notion that professionals from these two fields "have the resources to enable them to die at home, which suggests that financial concerns and lack of caregiver availability may be barriers to dying at home for less educated and affluent patients."[24]

Third, midcareer physicians simply know too much about the grim realities of dying to want their own deaths to look the way their patients' do. Their own experience caring for the most vulnerable and most ill patients forever alters the way they view their own mortality. This shift is unavoidable, really, when doctors spend years and years witnessing trauma being inflicted on their patients every day. It doesn't happen right when they graduate from medical school, or even within the first ten years of their practice. On the other side of the coin are the individual consumers, for whom this landscape is all new. They don't know that at the very best, this kind of treatment will extend their life by only a little bit, without improving its quality at all, and that at the end they will die anyway and their family and caregivers will be miserable.

Holly Prigerson, senior author and codirector of the Center for Research on End-of-Life Care at Weill Cornell, perfectly sums up this dichotomy: "When doctors themselves are facing death, they avoid intensive medical care, which we can assume is due to their knowledge of just how violent and futile those efforts typically are."[25] Yet if *violent* and *futile* are the words that are, ironically, associated with purportedly lifesaving efforts, shouldn't patients know what their doctors know? Shouldn't they, too, be allowed to die at home, in a peaceful, nonclinical environment, where ample pain management and hospice services are available to them? Shouldn't they have their advance care planning done so that they control their own outcomes? Certainly, few among us would consciously choose to undergo such physical and emotional rigors if we knew the outcome would be death anyway.

FINAL THOUGHTS

Something is amiss in the health care system. No better evidence of that exists than the fact that doctors themselves are choosing to die in ways that are very different from the ways in which they are allowing their patients to die. Palliative care delivered at home should be the standard for all people with a chronic, terminal, or complex health condition—not just for cancer patients, not just for the most elderly or wealthy people, and not just for people in hospice—and advance care planning should be as standard a part of getting our affairs in order as creating a will or renewing a driver's license. In order for US society to get to a point where these circumstances are the norm, not the exception, for people of all ethnic, socioeconomic, geographical, age, and medical backgrounds, the health care industry has a lot more research and a lot more learning to do. Nobody has all the answers right now, including me; nobody knows the exact route to palliative care's mainstream success, because the field is still too fragmented and too new. However, knowing what the issues are and what directions the conversations need to go in is the first step toward success. I'm here to educate you as best I can, and I hope that as the public continues to be more and more aware of this issue, the questions I'm asking will inspire you to reflect and pose your own inquiries, to open lines of communication that help everyone achieve a common understanding of the palliative care landscape, and to take action when the time comes for you to take control of your own medical destiny.

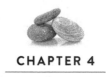

CHAPTER 4

How to Get the Care You Want

KNOWING WHAT TO ASK FOR, WHAT TO EXPECT, AND WHAT TO DEMAND

This is your world. Shape it, or someone else will.
—GARY LEW, FINANCIER

Do you know how you would want to be treated, medically, if you were seriously ill? Would you want a "pull out all the stops" approach (and do you even know what that means)? Have you shared that information with your family and your primary care physician? According to studies by the Centers for Disease Control and Prevention and many other reputable organizations, the answer is no. No, you haven't thought about what kind of medical care you would like; no, you do not understand what "life-prolonging care" means; and no, you have not discussed any of this with family members or your doctor. You may be part of a majority (approximately two-thirds of Americans fit this description), but it is not where you should want to be, particularly if you are fifty or older.[1]

The problem with a passive "head in the sand" attitude on this topic is that by default you will get care that most Americans, when surveyed, say they do *not* want: aggressive and, as we discussed in chapter 3, often futile treatments delivered by strangers in a loud, unpleasant environment, such as an intensive care unit or emergency room. Tethered to machines, possibly unable to speak because of intubation, stripped of a sense of self and dignity, and a universe away from the comforts of home—this is the common outcome for those who avoid thinking or talking about what kind of medical care they would want when faced with a medical crisis or serious illness. In most instances, you can be sure that you will *not* receive palliative care.

As earlier chapters have shown, doctors are highly unlikely to initiate a conversation about quality-of-life concerns because (1) they are focused on eradicating the disease at all costs, per their medical training, even when the diagnosis is terminal; (2) they are uncomfortable talking about the negative side effects of treatment; and (3) they are not trained to have these discussions.

You must be the one to start that dialogue. If you are facing chemotherapy, for example, tell your doctor you want palliative care concurrently. If you have a choice of agencies, ask your doctor for candid reviews of each. Even if you live in an isolated rural area, telemedicine for palliative care is often available; ask about that too.

This chapter makes it clear that you, the patient, have a say in your medical care. It empowers you to go to your health care appointments feeling prepared, to know what rights you have as a patient and what questions to ask to get the care you want, to identify a patient advocate, to understand what paperwork is important to have on hand, and to navigate hospitalization and discharge. It also supplies you with areas of potential concerns to consider and explains why you need to bring along a friend or family member to act as your patient advocate.

KNOW YOUR RIGHTS

On June 22, 2010, President Barack Obama, in conjunction with the Departments of Health and Human Services, Labor, and Treasury, released the Patient's Bill of Rights—a list of guarantees to anyone seeking treatment in a health care facility that empowers them to make decisions about their medical care, that does not discriminate against anyone with a preexisting condition who is seeking health insurance, and that protects individual privacy.[2]

But before Obamacare came into being, there was another Patient's Bill of Rights, this one by the American Hospital Association (AHA), introduced in 1973 and revised in 1992. This bill was established "with the expectation that it will contribute to more effective patient care and be supported by the hospital on behalf of the institution, its medical staff, employees, and patients," and the AHA "encourages health care institutions to tailor [it] to their patient community by translating and/or simplifying the language of this bill of rights as may be necessary to ensure that patients and their families understand their rights and responsibilities."[3] It provides "a foundation for understanding and respecting the rights and responsibilities of patients, their families, physicians, and other caregivers." The bill also encourages hospitals to "ensure a health care ethic that respects the role of patients in decision making about treatment choices and other aspects of their care" and to "be sensitive to cultural, racial, linguistic, religious, age, gender, and other differences, as well as the needs of persons with disabilities."[4] The bill's nine most salient points are detailed below. It's a long list, but all of this information is important to know *before* you are admitted to a hospital. The more educated you are as a consumer, the more control you will have over your care.

1. "The patient has the right to considerate and respectful care."

2. "The patient has the right to . . . relevant, current, and understandable information concerning diagnosis, treatment, and prognosis." (And if you need more information, you should ask for educational material.)[5]

3. "Except in emergencies when the patient lacks decision-making capacity and the need for treatment is urgent, the patient is entitled to . . . discuss and request information related to the specific procedures and/or treatments, the risks involved, the possible length of recuperation, and the medically reasonable alternatives and their accompanying risks and benefits."

4. "Patients have the right to know the identity of physicians, nurses, and others involved in their care, as well as when those involved are students, residents, or other trainees."

5. "The patient has the right to make decisions about the plan of care prior to and during the course of treatment and to refuse a recommended treatment or plan of care to the extent permitted by law and hospital policy and to be informed of the medical consequences of this action. In case of such refusal, the patient is entitled to other appropriate care and services that the hospital provides or transfer to another hospital." (In the context of palliative care, this means you could, for example, decline curative treatment altogether or choose palliative care to occur concurrently with curative treatment. You should make this decision when you are still well enough to be sound of mind and body.)

6. "The patient has the right to have an advance directive (such as a living will, health care proxy, or durable power of attorney for health care) concerning treatment or designating a surrogate decision-maker with the expectation that the hospital will honor the intent of that directive to the extent permitted by law and hospital policy."

7. "The patient has the right to every consideration of privacy."

8. "The patient has the right to expect reasonable continuity of care when appropriate and to be informed by physicians and other caregivers of available and realistic patient care options when hospital care is no longer appropriate."

9. "The patient has the right to be informed of hospital policies and practices that relate to patient care, treatment, and responsibilities . . . [and] of available resources for resolving disputes, grievances, and conflicts."[6]

GET EDUCATED

I can't emphasize this enough: *You*—not your doctor, not a hospital, not anyone else—should be in charge of decisions about your own physical, emotional, and spiritual well-being when you're facing a serious illness. Even if you're working with one of the biggest medical gurus out there, if you have questions, you need to ask them—as often as you need to—and if your doctor's judgment doesn't seem right, you must not hesitate to question that, either. Bring a list of questions to every one of your doctor visits—doing so saves time and is more efficient—and be aware that one of your patient rights is the right to question a doctor whenever you want. And remember, when you're ill, the doctor works for you, not the other way around. You don't need to be aggressive about it, but people are often intimidated by doctors, especially the ones with big names, and then sell themselves short by not being inquisitive enough.

The issue with patients who are timid is that doctors are often all too willing to step in and "play God." Paul Duberstein, chair of the health behavior, society, and policy department at Rutgers School of Public Health and author of a study called "Physician and Patient Characteristics Associated with More Intensive End-of-Life Care," says, "Some physicians are very

comfortable taking over the decision-making for their terminally ill patients. . . . [And] when physicians do take charge of
treatment decisions, patients are more likely to receive aggressive interventions at the end of life. As a result, patients end up
in intensive care units or emergency rooms in the days before
death, even though most people would rather die peacefully
at home."[7] If this information about the status quo were more
widely available to the public, people might think twice about
waffling over their medical choices. This is why you must be
educated on what might be coming up in your treatment plan
and on the importance of making decisions early in your treatment. Even in the event that you lack decision-making capacity,
are legally incompetent, or are a minor, someone else—a designated health care proxy or surrogate decision maker—can
exercise your patient rights for you, as item number 7 in the list
above indicates. If you're young and healthy, you may be reluctant to make any big decisions about your late-in-life plans; at
the very least, though, you should delegate a health care proxy
who will know what you want when the time comes.

In her book *The Patient's Checklist: 10 Simple Hospital Checklists to Keep You Safe, Sane, and Organized*, Elizabeth Bailey offers
a number of excellent suggestions to patients who may need a
pep talk in order to be their own best advocates. These include:

- You have to be an educated consumer. Don't be passive;
  take responsibility.

- You need to understand why every single action is being
  done to your body in the hospital.

- You need to agree that every action is necessary and
  appropriate treatment for you.

- You need to be sure that every detail of treatment is meant
  for you; this includes questioning the nature, dosage, and
  timing of any medication you are prescribed.

- Communication should be your number one priority—the hospital environment is hectic, with many disciplines working together and an enormous amount of information being shared. Check to make sure they are all communicating with one another (65 percent of adverse reactions are due to communication errors; an adverse reaction equals an unintended medical event).

- You need to be an active decision maker or have a family member actively involved in your care.

- Discuss your goals of care with your care team—what is important to you; what your values and wishes are.[8]

Of course, this kind of communication can be daunting for even the most self-confident and articulate patients, particularly amid the overwhelming knowledge that the end of their life may occur earlier than they expected. Especially early after your diagnosis, you might find yourself feeling overburdened with information, as if you're in a fog, and able to absorb only a small amount of it. It could take weeks to fully comprehend what you are going through. *This is normal.* So don't be embarrassed or uncomfortable about asking questions you have asked before. When David was diagnosed with leukemia, his doctor spent two hours going over the disease and everything we were going to face. I retained only 5 percent, at best, of what she said, and I had to ask her to rehash everything after the fact. It takes patience for a health care provider to give a bad diagnosis, because it often simply doesn't sink in the first time.

Having a patient advocate—a family member, friend, or palliative care expert—present for this kind of difficult discussion with your care team offers numerous benefits. Invite someone you trust to accompany you, and ask that person to take notes throughout the meeting or, with your doctor's permission, make an audio/video recording of the conversation, even if you are doing so yourself. Encourage your advocate to ask their own questions if they think a point needs clarification. That way, even if you have follow-up questions, you've done thorough record keeping along the way. You also have a witness to your experience, someone whom you can ask, "Did you hear what I was hearing?" or "When the doctor said this, how did you interpret it?" In addition, your advocate may be able to share observations about your mental health that you can't articulate yourself: "This is frightening. I'm depressed. This is taking away some of my favorite things I used to do that made my life meaningful." When you have someone else who can beat that drum for you, your doctor is more likely to grasp the importance of being proactive about your emotional well-being, by saying, "I'm going to refer you to a counselor, and I want you to follow up, even if you don't think you need it." That one referral can be a gateway to all kinds of other introductions to experts who can further ease your pain. But you're not likely to reach that level of care if you don't ask for what you need.

HOW TO GET PALLIATIVE CARE

As you know by now, to gain access to palliative care, you will have to ask your doctor for it directly, but if you find yourself in the position of needing it, the following specific points, courtesy of GetPalliativeCare.org, will help you to facilitate the conversation:

- Tell your doctor you are thinking about palliative care, and ask where palliative care is available in your area.

- Ask your doctor to explain your illness and any past, current, and future treatments and procedures.

- Explain to your doctor exactly what quality of life means to you. This list may include being able to spend time with

loved ones, wanting relief from any pain and other symptoms; having the ability to make your own decisions for care
and where you want to be treated (home vs. in the hospital).

• Be sure your doctor is aware of any personal, religious, or
cultural beliefs, values, or practices that are important to
consider in your care and treatment decisions.

• Tell your doctor which treatments you may or may not want.

• Mention that you would like time to discuss future planning
for your care. You should do this even if you're well or it's
early in your illness.

• If you have completed a living will or health care proxy, be
sure to tell your doctor and provide him or her with a copy.

• Finally, at any point in your illness if you are experiencing
symptoms and stress, ask your doctor for the palliative care
referral![9]

Take a list of these and any other questions you have to
meetings with your health care providers, and do not hesitate to
ask any of them. Everyone has different priorities that pertain
to their health and any medical conditions they have, and the
more you can share your individual concerns with your doctor,
the more likely you are to get the support you're seeking.

ESSENTIAL PAPERWORK

Another aspect of being prepared if you or a loved one becomes
seriously ill is having your paperwork in order. These documents
include your birth certificate; marriage license; property titles
and list of assets; retirement planning, tax planning, financial planning, and estate planning documents; and a power of

attorney document. In addition, you should have a living will, which specifies what kind of life-sustaining medical intervention (tube feeding, ventilator, cardiopulmonary resuscitation [CPR]) you would want if you were to become terminally ill and/or permanently incapacitated.

I also can't recommend highly enough that you keep a journal or notebook filled with the most up-to-date medical information that you may want to discuss with your doctor if you are hospitalized. It should contain a list of any medications you're on (names, dosages, schedules), your vital information (date of birth, Social Security number, health insurance information), any allergies you have, and your primary care physician's name and contact information. Keep it with you at all times, in case you are hospitalized unexpectedly. When David was having severe complications from his stem cell transplant, he developed a rash, and his care team was concerned that it was going to internalize and affect his stomach and other organs in his body. They decided after several weeks to immunosuppress him. They gave him a large dose of prednisone before they discharged him, and one day after we got home, I heard him fall and found him having a seizure. The paramedics came and took him to the emergency room at our local hospital. When the ER doctor asked me, "Can you tell me what medication he's on?" I had my journal with me and gave him the complete list. The doctor turned white before my eyes. It was obvious that this was an overwhelming amount of information and that he and his staff lacked knowledge of David's treatment history. Then, when they physically assessed David, they noticed the bruises all over his body caused by his medications. When they saw those bruises, they were ready to call in social services because they actually thought we were physically abusing David. Finally, one of the nurses said she would vouch for our character because her son and daughter were in David's class. She said she knew us personally and knew that David was going through cancer treatment.

That incident was an important lesson for us. Most people believe that when they go to a doctor and tell him, "I have a pain somewhere inside me that can't be seen from the outside," the doctor will know everything about them just by looking in their eyes. But that's simply not the case. So when you come without any supporting information about your situation, no matter how much of an emergency it is, health care providers start from scratch. They start from "What's your name, and who's your medical insurance provider?" The point is, don't assume that doctors know anything about you (they don't), and don't assume that medical teams don't make mistakes (they do, all the time). It's your responsibility to help make sure they don't make those mistakes with you.

HOSPITALIZATION AND DISCHARGE

If you do end up in the hospital with a serious illness, the experience can be daunting, but there are concrete steps you can take to make the process smoother for yourself, both while you're there and after you're discharged. Slidell Memorial Hospital offers the following tips to help patients avoid becoming overwhelmed before and during their hospital stay:

- Get your paperwork in order: Ask hospital staff and your surgeon, if applicable, what forms you can fill out before you're admitted. Bring your Social Security card, photo ID, and insurance card to the hospital with you.

- Print your medical records: "Talk with your primary care physician and make sure your medical records are current. The hospital should be able to reference those documents during your stay, but don't assume everything was sent. Bring a printed copy of your medical file, including medical directive documents (including a living will and durable power of attorney), a list of all medications you're currently taking, any allergies you may have and contact information for your regular doctors."[10]

• Know where you're going: Ask about parking ahead of time, and use the on-site maps to guide you once you're inside the hospital.

• Keep asking questions: Being proactive and inquisitive will help you get the best care possible. In a *Huffington Post* article, Dr. Jim Merino, chief experience officer at the Cleveland Clinic, says, "Don't stop [asking questions] until you have a complete understanding of the experience." Doctors are "dealing with people in the worst possible situation of their lives," he adds. "They're fearful; they have anxiety and uncertainty. If a caregiver gets offended, those patients should find a different physician."[11] Remember, you can't assume that your care team knows everything about your condition and your treatment unless you talk to them about it.

• Take copious notes: Keep a notebook handy, and write down the name and other identifying details of anyone who comes into your room, gives you medications, or tells you anything about your care. When you're amid a seemingly endless parade of people coming and going, and especially if you're taking mind-altering medications, you'll need this record to serve as your memory. Also take notes on how you're responding to medications and other treatment protocols. For example, no matter what specific condition you have, doctors will bring up certain lab values again and again in conversation with you. If you have cancer, they'll ask about your platelets all the time. If you have an issue with blood pressure, they'll check your blood pressure more often. If you're diabetic, they'll want to know your blood-sugar levels. Every time someone walks into your room and asks, "What was the patient's last platelet count?" you save time if you've already written it down and can say, "The number this morning was . . ." The more familiar with medical lingo you can become, the better off you'll be, and the more time you'll save your health care providers.[12]

If you are a religious or spiritual person, you may have certain preferences that could affect your care. For example, a patient's beliefs often impact the medical decisions they make. In addition, religions have a bearing on choices about diet, modesty, and the preferred gender of a patient's health providers. Also, some religions have strict prayer times that may interfere with medical treatment.[13] If you need guidance in these areas or any other, ask to speak with a hospital chaplain, social worker, or caseworker. These trained professionals have a responsibility to listen to and respect patients' individual faith-based wishes, and to tailor their treatment accordingly.

After you address all of these considerations, you'll want to think about what happens when you're ready to be discharged. You'll no doubt be eager to get home, but it behooves you to take your time with this process as well. It may involve final tests or lab procedures, and a nurse should give you instructions regarding follow-up visits and any medications you'll need. However, just because you're leaving the hospital doesn't mean you're out of time to ask questions—on the contrary, this is a crucial period in which to get as much information as you need to feel comfortable going home. A few important considerations to cover with your care team are:

- Are your family members/caregivers aware of what you'll need after discharge? What should you and they expect after hospitalization—in terms of mobility, self-care, changes in appetite, anxiety, and so forth?

- Do you feel as if you're being discharged too soon? If so, you can appeal your discharge.

- Do you know what parts of your hospitalization and treatment your health insurance will and will not cover? Gather as much information as you can about your financial obligations (co-pays and out-of-pocket expenses).

- What questions do you have about any instructions you were given regarding your medications, diet, exercise, medical equipment you will need at home, and activities to avoid?

- When should you follow up with your doctors? When is your next appointment? Whom should you contact in case of an emergency?

The discharge stage is one in which palliative care is particularly relevant and useful. First, most patients who are being discharged will receive some type of medication for pain. This medicine isn't intended to heal them; it's meant simply to mask symptoms and make people more comfortable. By definition, that step of discharge falls under the umbrella of palliative care.

Second, and more important, patients who receive a long checklist of things to do after a hospitalization often become overwhelmed. When you're receiving post-hospitalization directions, a palliative care social worker can help organize all this information on your behalf. One of their jobs when someone leaves the hospital is to have that checklist in hand, to know when and how the patient should carry it out, and to know when to follow up with the patient. This last item is becoming more and more relevant as a movement toward palliative care in outpatient settings gains more and more traction. Instead of having to receive palliative care services at a hospital, where the risk of getting some kind of infection is much higher, patients can receive the same care from the comfort of their home or a state-of-the-art outpatient clinic.

This new model of care benefits everyone. Today, hospitals, doctors, and especially insurance companies want to get patients home as soon as possible, because doing so decreases their chance of injury or infection. Therefore, it stands to reason that if we can keep patients out of the hospitals in the first place while still helping them to feel better, not to mention cutting costs for everyone, outpatient palliative care is a win-win. Already, a variety of health care facilities are rallying for the cause, including Beth Israel Deaconess Medical Center in Massachusetts, the University of New Mexico Hospital, Baylor Scott & White Health in Texas, and Hospice and Community Care in Pennsylvania.[14] In addition, as of 2021, the Accreditation Commission for Health Care (ACHC) offers accreditation for community-based providers who provide in-home palliative care.[15] Ideally, once a patient is discharged from the hospital (or even before they ever have to enter one), they will continue to reap the advantages of this burgeoning trend.

FINAL THOUGHTS

You've probably heard the saying "Knowledge is power." Now that you understand that you may not be able to rely on your doctors to be proactive about giving you all the information you need to receive the best possible medical, emotional, and spiritual care, you need to gain that knowledge on your own. That is what will make you a powerful champion of your own well-being. My intention in writing this chapter is to encourage you to inhabit that power—by never being afraid to speak up; by never hesitating to ask questions (and then to ask them again if you don't get the answers you want the first time); and by being courageous enough to challenge the health care industry as a whole to be more successful at its purported mission to help sick and injured people feel better so that they can enjoy life. These are not just your rights; they're your responsibility—to medical experts, to your family and friends, and, most of all, to yourself.

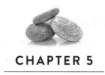

CHAPTER 5

How to Cope When Illness Changes Everything

QUALITY-OF-LIFE CARE INCLUDES THE FAMILY

When the unthinkable happens, the lighthouse is hope.
Once we choose hope, everything is possible.
—CHRISTOPHER REEVE (1952–2004), ACTOR, DIRECTOR, AND ACTIVIST

From age five to age ten—the very heart of her childhood—our daughter, Sarah, lived in the shadow of David's battle with cancer. Joe and I each had special duties in caring for David, and when Sarah expressed interest in participating, she became part of David's "team" as well.

After David's stem cell transplant, he was not able to eat, and he had a gastric tube inserted in his stomach to provide nourishment that he could not tolerate receiving in the traditional way. Preparing his liquid meals was a relatively simple task, so I taught Sarah how to open the container of formula and pour it into the bag that supplied the feeding tube attached to David's stomach. In addition, when David relapsed after his stem cell transplant, he couldn't have visitors because he was immunosuppressed. That was another area where Sarah really shone as a caregiver: she was his only playmate. Even though there was a six-year difference between them, he depended on her for much of his social interaction. She embraced these responsibilities as part of our family's collective effort to conquer the disease that had taken over our lives.

A serious illness affects not just the patient but every member of that person's family. Routines are shattered, anxieties about the ill loved one obliterate normal activities, and each member of a family suffers in a unique way. Men and women cope differently, and children do too. At a time when you need one another more than ever, the circumstances of an illness can drive a wedge between even the strongest of parent partnerships and parent-child relationships.

This chapter offers down-to-earth guidance as you and your family navigate this new territory. One tactic is including everyone in the family care team, but many others are available to you as well, particularly through palliative care. As we've discussed, palliative care's focus is on quality of life for the seriously ill or injured person; however, it also recognizes that how well a family copes with a life-threatening illness affects the patient profoundly and that the well-being of that person's family members matters too, since their state of mind affects the patient, and vice versa. No matter how many studies show that patients want to be *home*, if that environment is fraught with tension because you are overcome by the difficulty of the disease, your loved one may suffer from feeling like a burden.

This chapter also helps your caregivers to realize that it's okay to ask for help for *themselves*, and to tap into what palliative care can offer in that regard. How they cope during a loved one's illness will also affect how they cope if that condition leads to death; their thoughts and actions during these weeks and months are an essential part of what might be the most meaningful and poignant experience of their life.

EMOTIONAL DISTRESS

An abundance of literature about the mind-body-spirit connection exists today, but that concept takes on a whole new meaning when a serious illness is involved. When you receive a diagnosis, everything that your body is going through can suddenly translate into a flood of emotions that feel like ocean waves, crashing over you again and again, each one not quite like the last or the next. You may be shocked or numb. You may be worried or terrified. You may feel profoundly sad and helpless. According to HelpGuide, other common emotional responses to serious illness may include:

• Anger or frustration as you struggle to come to terms with your diagnosis—repeatedly asking, "Why me?" or trying to understand if you've done something to deserve this.

• Facing up to your own mortality and the prospect that the illness could potentially be life-ending.

• Worrying about the future—how you'll cope, how you'll pay for treatment, what will happen to your loved ones, the pain you may face as the illness progresses, or how your life may change.

• Grieving the loss of your health and old life.

• Feeling powerless, hopeless, or unable to look beyond the worst-case scenario.

• Regret or guilt about things you've done that you think may have contributed to your illness or injury. Shame at how your condition is affecting those around you.

• Denial that anything is wrong or refusing to accept the diagnosis.

• A sense of isolation, feeling cut off from friends and loved ones who can't understand what you're going through.

• A loss of self. You're no longer you but rather your medical condition.[1]

While every one of these thoughts and feelings is normal and valid at a time like this—and in fact may also reflect the way some caregivers, not just patients, feel about an illness in their midst—you must promise yourself to be hands-on at identifying and relying on coping mechanisms if you find yourself emotionally overwhelmed, let alone descending into full-blown clinical anxiety or depression.

COPING MECHANISMS FOR PATIENTS AND CAREGIVERS

The good news is, whether you're a patient or a caregiver, there's no shortage of ways to get the support you need to handle your new reality. HelpGuide and Vistas Healthcare provide excellent summaries of the most productive means of doing so.

1. Reach out for support.
   - Choose the support that's right for you.
   - Don't let worries about being a burden keep you from reaching out.
   - Look for support from friends and loved ones who are good listeners.
   - Make face time a priority.
   - Join a support group.
   - Seek out a peer support program.

2. Explore your emotions.
   - Give yourself permission to experience all of your feelings fully, even if they scare you. You don't have to pretend to act positive and upbeat if you don't feel that way.
   - If you are experiencing negative emotions, own them. You will only benefit yourself by being honest about the way you're feeling. Venting frustration is healthier than keeping it bottled up and can ultimately help you to feel stronger and more equipped to manage your illness.

3. Manage stress.
   • Talk to someone you trust.
   • Adopt a relaxation practice.
   • Get enough sleep.
   • Be as active as possible.

4. Pursue activities that bring you meaning and joy.
   • Pick up a long-neglected hobby.
   • Learn something new.
   • Get involved in your community.
   • Spend time in nature.
   • Enjoy the arts.
   • Write a memoir.

5. Deal with anxiety and depression.
   • Manage debilitating symptoms, such as pain.
   • Ease up on the worrying.
   • Take care of yourself.
   • Cut down on sugar in your diet.
   • Be smart about caffeine, alcohol, and nicotine.
   • Accept uncertainty.[2]

6. Try alternative therapies.[3]
   • Psychotherapy, occupational therapy, reiki, acupuncture, biofeedback, nutritional counseling, aromatherapy, animal therapy, art or music therapy, massage—you name it—have been shown to quantifiably improve seriously ill patients' quality of life.

CAREGIVERS: FAMILY MATTERS

As of 2021, more than forty-eight million Americans were caregivers for a family member or friend. Although many of those caregivers provide that service at no charge, all fifty US states now offer patients self-directed Medicaid services for long-term care. This means that individuals can qualify to manage their own home care—and in some states, that includes designating a family member as a paid caregiver. Former military service members are entitled to the same benefit.[4]

Compensated or not, family members can always find ways to support an ill patient. Listening quietly, vocalizing your availability to support the patient as needed, educating yourself about the patient's illness but not giving advice unless the patient asks for it, and generally staying connected are all easy, helpful tactics to employ.

Other times, support extends into the physical realm, whether you're bathing the patient, taking them for walks or to medical appointments, or providing meals. In our case, physical assistance extended even further, to extreme sacrifice, when we found out that David had to have a stem cell transplant and that his sister, Sarah, was his closest donor match. David wanted to be sure that Sarah did not feel any pressure to donate her stem cells, as she was only nine years old at the time. But when we explained it to her, as much as you can explain anything like that to a child that age, even though we were honest with her that it was not going to be a pleasant experience, she didn't hesitate to volunteer.

After she agreed, I had to give her shots for several days to boost her white cell count, and then she had to get a catheter put in her leg because the doctors needed a large artery to take out her blood. Then she had to go to a blood receiving room and spend two days hooked up to a machine that harvested her stem cells. She drew a picture of the experience and was very proud of the fact that she was doing something so special for David.

David was, of course, very appreciative. He thanked her officially, but then one day shortly before the transplant, he said to us, "I need to go to the bank." Joe went with him. He had a savings account and withdrew some money from it. When Joe asked what he was going to do with it, he said, "We need to go to a jewelry store—I want to buy Sarah a gold chain." He and his sister had a deep bond from the beginning, but when he was ill, it got even stronger. When family members treat the individual's illness as a problem to tackle together, the emotional rewards can be boundless.

That doesn't mean siblings of children with cancer or other life-threatening illnesses have it easy. On the contrary, these kids are often not a priority in the general scheme of things; they are sometimes forgotten and many times may become jealous of attention that their ill sibling is receiving from well-meaning people. In the worst-case scenarios, says one study,

> Having a sibling with chronic disease constitutes a risk for psychological health and well-being in children. It . . . renders them more susceptible to mental diseases and weaker psychosocial functions, and these effects also continue in adulthood. Many problems, including anxiety, depression, symptoms of posttraumatic stress, lower quality of life values, and/or peer problems may be observed in these children. . . . These children may overreact to changes in family life, experience separation anxiety, and think that they are outside the family order. . . . As a result, families may fail to satisfy the needs of the other siblings because they mostly focus on the child who is sick. Healthy siblings may potentially become forgotten, disregarded, and neglected children.[5]

In her seminal book, *On Children and Death*, renowned psychiatrist Elisabeth Kübler-Ross discusses this same phenomenon, explaining,

> Many brothers and sisters have responded with increasing negativity to their terminally ill siblings when parents react to the illness with excessive pampering. We have

innumerable cases where the sick child was treated like
a hero, where famous people were asked to write or visit
them, where gifts and privileges were given to them far
in abundance of anything the siblings could ever hope
to receive. With parental guilt and overindulgence, it is
no surprise when many of the brothers and sisters start
acting out.[6]

If you have multiple children and find yourself in a situation
like the ones above, please seek psychological counseling as soon
as possible, both for your sick child's sibling(s) and for yourself
as parents. Nipping these potential issues in the bud is critical for your entire family's well-being, and for your children's
future. If you do your due diligence in this regard, you may find
that your well children still exhibit some behavioral or attitudi-
nal challenges, but you'll have a better chance of mitigating any
really damaging long-term consequences.

Sarah never complained or expressed jealousy while David
was alive, but even she eventually acknowledged having felt
like number two for a long time. After David died, we moved
to Hampstead, in London. When we toured our house for the
first time, we looked at all the bedrooms upstairs. I wanted to
put Sarah in the smaller of two rooms, but she said, "For years,
I didn't complain about things, but right now, I want the larger
room." It was a nice way to let us know that she was aware of the
fact that David was no longer with us. It also made me realize
that I hadn't yet adjusted to the fact that we had lost him. Part
of me was thinking, *This bigger bedroom would have been David's*.
Sarah had to be the one to say, "Well, David's not here anymore,
so it's my turn." And she was absolutely right. It was her way of
standing up for herself after all that time and asking for something that would give her a better quality of life at home.

If you are the parent of a sick child, quality of life should be a
priority for you as well, no matter how distracting or exhausting

your role as a caregiver may feel sometimes. Two of the best things you can do to ease your burdens are to (1) ask friends and other supportive figures for help and (2) reprioritize your life. I had to learn to say no to future commitments—an art unto itself. You simply can't "do it all" when you're trying to parent two or more children and one of them is sick and/or hospitalized.

Through my experience with David, I learned that I'm very good at helping others and very bad at asking for help myself. It took me a long time to get comfortable with reaching out to people, but when I did, I learned that they really *wanted* to help. My mother, who died of a degenerative neurological disease in 2008, was the same way—she was always there to help others, but once she got sick, she had a hard time asking for what she needed. I had gained some valuable insights by then from taking care of David, and I remember saying to her, "You know what, Mom? One thing I've discovered is that your friends want so much to help and to show you how much they care about you. All you have to do is allow them to come into your world a little bit, and you will be amazed at how much love you will receive if you allow it to happen."

I'll never forget when David was first diagnosed with leukemia and I came home from the hospital one day to find that someone I didn't even know had come by my house and fully stocked my refrigerator. I couldn't believe someone had done that for me, let alone a stranger. It was such an incredible experience, so humbling, to be on the receiving end of that gesture. As time goes by and you start accepting little bits of what people are providing you, through meals or spending time with your child, you'll realize that the secondary gain is how much love you receive—love that you're used to giving to other people. That was one of the lifelong lessons I learned from David: Yes, we should always strive to be good to others, but people also want to be good to us. Don't deny the people who want to help you. Instead, simply open your arms and say, "Thank you so much!"

In addition to our remarkable support network, the four of us as a family all fueled each other. When one of us was low, another person would pick us up. Most of the time, because David was still a child, he reacted to however Joe and I were responding to a situation. As long as he saw that Joe and I were supporting each other and in control and laughing with him, he never thought too far ahead; he just dealt with things one day at a time. But these situations go both ways, so his emotional state had a real impact on us as well. In the very beginning, especially after the first round of chemo and after his stem cell transplant, there were days when he just felt awful. He'd come downstairs in the morning, and whatever his mood was would tell me how my day was going to go. If he was in a great mood, then my whole day was great. On a bad day, we all just did our best to get through it. I was listening to a lot of South American music during that time, and whenever David's mood got really bad I did one of two things—either I played my South American music and danced around the house, or I howled with our family dogs. I had two dogs, and every time an ambulance or a fire truck went by, the dogs would start howling with the sirens. Soon we'd all join in, and the dogs would keep going along with us. Howling was the way our family broke our cycle of despair. It was very primal. That was another important piece of wisdom David shared with us: you have to enter a period of illness as a family, and everyone has their own role to play and contributions to make. No matter what, you have to work together.

Other coping mechanisms that our family found helpful during David's illness included:

- Doing group activities that gave us a sense of normalcy, such as watching TV together, playing games, going outdoors, playing with our pets, and going for drives.

- Reminiscing about our happy times together—favorite vacations and other special moments.

• Encouraging extended family and friends to visit us, if they were allowed (when David was not immuno-suppressed).

• Developing new hobbies together, such as singing, painting, journaling, and writing.

• Finding solace in simple pleasures, which, we discovered, brought us joy and connected us as a family much more deeply than we had been before David was ill; life became precious, and we all realized that you have to seize the moment (carpe diem).

• Encouraging David to do as much as possible for himself, even though he may not have felt up to it—for example, we paid him to babysit Sarah—so that we could give him a sense of responsibility, pride, and accomplishment.

MARITAL CHALLENGES AND ADVICE

It seems shocking to think about now, but prior to David's illness, Joe and I had some marital issues. Fortunately, we went to a therapist and realized that we wanted the same things out of life, so, by the time David got sick, we were back on solid ground and we knew we were going to be there for each other, no matter what. Still, David was traumatized by our separation. I remember that when he was home after his first round of chemo, he was feeling awful and I was in nurse mode, wanting to help him. When I asked him, "What can I do to make you feel comfortable?" he said, "Mom, I just want to be a family." That, to him, was the most important thing to focus on.

When a child is in the midst of a medical crisis, even the strongest partnerships can be tested. Coparents have less time to nurture their own relationship than they typically do, because all of their energy shifts to caring for their child and handling their many other day-to-day responsibilities. As a result, if the couple has any issues before the child is diagnosed, they will almost certainly come to a head during the illness. In fact, when David was going through cancer treatment, some of the psychologists we came into contact with were studying how parents cope after a complex procedure like a stem cell transplant. They kept telling us that the majority of their patients' parents would eventually divorce because the experience of having a sick child just tore their marriages apart. Joe and I were among the lucky ones who stayed together and who continue to be married—we celebrated our fortieth anniversary in 2021—but that's partly because we happened to do the work of seeing a couples' counselor before he was diagnosed.

So many mothers and fathers have totally different ways of coping with an illness, and that sometimes works against them. We saw evidence of this contrast when David was undergoing treatment at Memorial Sloan Kettering: the mothers were always by the bedside, never getting a break, and the fathers were off at work. This was not the case for Joe and me. Instead, I was with David during the day and Joe was with him at night. Then Joe went to work during the day and I went home at night to manage our household and take care of Sarah. Throughout that arrangement, Joe and I were consistent about dividing our time with David equally, and we always kept our line of communication open. We also found small ways to spend time together, just the two of us. Most often, when I showed up at the hospital in the morning to relieve Joe after he'd spent all night with David, we'd go to a coffee shop across the street and have breakfast together. Simple efforts like that in a time of crisis can go a long way toward keeping a couple's bond strong. Having a sick child can break a lot of couples, but it can also be the glue that holds them together. It just depends on their dynamic and their willingness to do whatever they need to do to be a unified front. Whether during the illness, during the treatment, or after the child passes away, the most important thing is that parents work together as a team.

It was never lost on Joe and me that we were financially in a place many other people weren't. We had a nice, comfortable home, close to the hospital, and we had top-notch medical insurance through Joe's job as an executive at a worldwide financial institution. Our struggles were nothing in comparison with some of the other families we met. We encountered a lot of people at the hospital who didn't have the same means we did, who came from other countries, or who had to live separately because the husband was working two jobs to make ends meet and the mother had to keep their children with her.

During that time, I also discovered the extent of the stress that trying to navigate medical insurance can cause. We got to know many other families when David was first diagnosed and we were going to the oncologist's office all the time. I sat in that room with the other sick kids' parents every week and was blown away by how many of them were struggling to get their health insurance companies to pay for their children's chemotherapy. Our family was fortunate not to have to face that particular obstacle, but these other families' experiences inspired me to write to one of our Connecticut state senators and talk to him about how many of them were battling not only for their child's health but also for their insurance companies to pay for the treatments.

If you are struggling to cover your child's medical costs, talk to your hospital's finance department or consult a financial advisor. Also, look into organizations like Ronald McDonald House, which gives some parents free housing when their child is in the hospital, and hospitals like St. Jude, where you can take a child for cancer treatment free of charge and which helps parents with accommodations and other basic needs.

Financial troubles are always hard, but when they are paired with a significant illness, they can become unbearable. Money troubles or disagreements over money are widely known to be one of the top causes of divorce in the United States, even for couples who *don't* have a sick child. Add a bunch of red tape and a sick child to the equation, and it's no wonder marital strife arises. And how do people cope with all this incredible stress? Many of them drink to excess, have extramarital affairs, or simply check out and stop communicating with their partner altogether. These behaviors only lead to more marital discord. This vicious cycle has to end if two estranged parents are to find their way back to each other. Engaging a therapist whose mission it is to bring people together during this trying time can make all the difference for some couples. Luckily for Joe and me, that happened before David's illness, so we were ready to stand up to it as one.

LAUGHTER: THE GREAT HEALER

When a loved one is ill, the temptation to cry, to ask why, or to live in fear of negative outcomes is powerful. But it doesn't have to be that way. One thing I learned from David is that whenever the going gets really tough, laughter truly is, as the saying goes, the best medicine. My son knew that better than anyone. There were so many times when, even in the midst of extreme suffering, he made himself and everyone around him laugh. It was his way of taking control of the cancer and, in some cases, even managing his pain and discomfort. During some of the most difficult moments, David would joke with Joe at night, when Joe was with him in the hospital, in order to keep the unpleasantness of his symptoms in check. He never missed an opportunity to jump on something that would give him and the rest of us some comic relief.

That started early on, even before David got sick. From a very young age, he could detect good humor easily in others and had excellent comedic timing. He and Joe joked around all the time. When he was undergoing chemo, he started losing his hair within a few weeks. When Joe, who was also balding, tried to make light of it, David, without batting an eye, shot back at Joe, "Yes, but mine will grow back in. Yours will not."

Another time, he turned a radiation session into a humorous situation. In preparation for his stem cell transplant, he had to have three weeks of chemotherapy, followed by several rounds of radiation. Each session of the latter took place in a sealed chamber—I'm talking about two-foot-thick cement walls.

David was tied to a contraption that left his arms sticking out to each side. He looked like he was being crucified. The only way for Joe and me to see him was through a video camera. It had a microphone, and just before they started the radiation, he asked Joe, "Dad, can you see me?"

Joe said, "Yes, David, I can see you."

His arms were open like that, and he tilted and lowered his head to one side and then asked, "Do I remind you of someone?" Imagine that—he was really sick, trapped inside a bunker, and the kid still had enough of a sense of humor to poke fun at himself.

Another of our favorite funny stories happened after the transplant, when David was in isolation. One Sunday, a performer from the Big Apple Circus in New York came to entertain the children. This guy came in and was all made up like a clown, with the crazy makeup and the big shoes and everything. He stuck his head in the door and said, "Hi, David."

David, still very weak, quietly motioned to the man and said, "Come a little closer."

The man asked, "Why? What is it you want to say?"

David said, "Who does your makeup?"

The man asked, "Why?"

David said, "You've got to get yourself somebody new, because you look like a clown."

The clown was in shock—I don't think he was used to having a kid who was so frail and so weak have such a quick wit—but we all laughed and laughed about it.

SUPPORT FOR CAREGIVERS

Former First Lady of the United States Rosalyn Carter once said, "There are only four kinds of people in the world: those who have been caregivers, those who are currently caregivers, those who will be caregivers, and those who will need caregivers." This quote has long resonated with me because I know firsthand how valuable a caregiver can be in improving quality of life for ill people. Not only have I been one myself, for David, but as a nurse and educator, I've witnessed this magic happen time and time again.

The definition of caregiving spans a wide variety of tasks, including personal care, mobility, transportation, communication, housework, management and coordination of medical care, administration of medications and therapies, emotional support, assistance with personal care, organizing appointments, social services, assistance with social activities, managing money, ambulating, transferring, incontinence care, shopping, housework, meal preparation, making telephone calls, and managing finances.[7] All too often, the sad outcome of shouldering so many responsibilities is that caregivers suffer as much as or even more than their patients do. In 2021, one group of researchers discovered that

> at the physical level, ICs [informal caregivers] experience challenges associated with assisting in physically strenuous daily activities of living. At the psychosocial level, ICs are more likely to experience higher levels of anxiety, depression, and social isolation than formal or non-caregivers.

At the economic level, ICs incurred significant out-of-pocket medical expenses. As the [patient's] disease(s) progress, ICs are often left with no choice but to reduce or to give up work entirely to provide care.[8]

As if those findings weren't sobering enough, in a revealing first-person article in the *Huffington Post* called "No One Gives a Rat's Ass about Family Caregivers," Ann Brenoff describes the eye-opening experience of becoming her ill husband's caregiver and discovering the hard way that although "caregivers save the government more than $500 billion a year by doing jobs that nurses and paid professionals should be doing . . . , anywhere from 30 percent to 70 percent of caregivers die before their patients" because the job is so stressful. She even goes so far as to say, "Caregivers are the most overwhelmed group of people I have ever encountered."[9]

If you are a caregiver and you find yourself feeling worn down, overburdened, anxious, or depressed, do not feel ashamed or reluctant to seek help. Although caregivers have "expressed interest in learning more about what to expect at every stage of their loved one's illness and how to manage behavioral changes and coexisting medical conditions and complications in their loved one," health care providers are as yet largely remiss in providing such information, even though they are uniquely positioned to spot caregiver burdens and to support caregivers either directly or through pointing them in the direction of helpful resources.[10] Fortunately, some initiatives—including the Family Caregiver Alliance, the National Institute on Aging, and the CARE Act—are stepping in to fill the void that the health care industry is currently creating in this area.

Although the benefits of palliative care are clear for people living with a serious illness, they can be just as valuable for care-givers to manage their own physical and emotional health. A good palliative care team is focused not just on helping patients understand their illness but also on teaching caregivers how to make informed decisions, prepare for the future, and match the patient's goals with treatment options. A social worker, case manager, or hospital staff members can help connect caregivers with community resources, such as meals and home health and transport needs, as well as caregiver support groups.[11] If no one on your patient's palliative care team offers you these options, *ask for them*. If you aren't practicing self-care—if you are tired, undernourished, overworked, confused about your role, or deprived of your own social life—you can't possibly provide the best possible care for your patients.

FINAL THOUGHTS

People who have a serious illness want their life to return to normal. They want to feel well enough to spend quality time with family and friends, rather than experiencing all of the emotional upheaval that typically accompanies a diagnosis and treatment. That wish may not be realistic, but in the space that former, familiar routines once filled, a new normal will eventually emerge—one in which palliative care can help anyone directly involved to feel comfortable. To that end, I hope you will take advantage of the guidance I've offered in this chapter. It has been my honor over the years to share insights from my family's journey through terminal illness with others who are now in the midst of the battle. The experience is never easy. It can be exhausting, divisive, infuriating. It will change you forever in ways that you can't anticipate now. But even in your darkest moments, even when you think you can't stand your situation for even one more day, I want you to know that you can. You can cope with more hardship than you could possibly realize when you're in the thick of it. It takes hard work and self-awareness, but ultimately you will cherish the benefits of putting in the time to help your family—the sick members *and* the well members—feel stable and supported. And you will not fail if you remember that there is *always* joy to be found in life, even when illness turns it upside down.

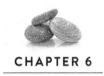

CHAPTER 6

Putting It All Together

CREATING AN ACTION PLAN FOR WHEN THE END IS NEAR

The bad news is, time flies.
The good news is, you're the pilot.
—MICHAEL ALTSHULER, MOTIVATIONAL SPEAKER

Most of us don't plan for the onset of a serious illness. Why would we? We're going to enjoy good health until an advanced old age and then die peacefully in our sleep. That picture, however, is not going to be the reality for the vast majority of us. As we discussed in chapter 3, most Americans die in hospitals, where doctors are treating them with extreme measures for life-ending illnesses. Yet national surveys consistently show that nearly 90 percent of us say we want to die at home.

The way to begin trying to address this disconnect is by answering a question that Angelo Volandes, MD (Harvard Medical School, Massachusetts General Hospital), asks: "How do you want to *live?*" Volandes is the author of the book *The Conversation*, which tells the stories of seven different seriously ill patients and the divergent paths their final experiences take, based on whether they do or do not have a conversation with their doctors about how they want to spend the rest of their lives. In Volandes's view, doctors' failure to ask and understand such patients' wishes is "the most urgent issue facing America today" and explains why "two-thirds of people age 65 or older end up dying in hospitals, often tethered to machines and in a good deal of pain."[1]

The good news is, if you do not want to be part of this sta-
tistic, you *can* avoid it—but only if you are willing to initiate a
conversation with your doctor. We need to talk about what we
want from health care should we fall seriously ill. Our wishes
should become a part of everyday discussions with our family
and friends, not a topic to be scared of but a topic to help us
understand how to live the best life. As Sunita Puri, palliative
medicine physician and author of the memoir *That Good Night:
Life and Medicine in the Eleventh Hour*, explains,

> Our collective silence about death, suffering and mortality
> places a tremendous burden on the people we love, and on
> the doctors and nurses navigating these conversations. We
> should not be discussing our loved one's wishes for the first
> time when they are in an ICU bed, voiceless and pinned
> in place by machines and tubes. Talking about death is
> ultimately talking about life—about who and what matters
> to us, and how we can live well even when we are dying.
> Rather than being motivated by fear and anxiety, we can
> open these discussions from a place of care and concern.[2]

This chapter provides a checklist and a wealth of down-to-
earth tactics to start this dialogue. You'll find detailed information on conversation starters and possible questions to ask,
concrete advice about advance care planning, and more.

Serious or terminal illness creates chaos and sorrow. While
you can't always avoid the sorrow, you can skip a lot of the chaos
if you have a good plan in place. That plan starts with a talk that
just might be the most important one you'll ever have.

AN ACTION PLAN

We'll go over all these ideas in more detail throughout this chapter, but the following list is a distilled version of the steps you'll

want to take to ensure that you have the best life possible in whatever time you have left—even if you still have decades to go.

1. The talk starts with a series of personal inquiries. Ask yourself what the elements of a joyful day are for you, and write down what you come up with. Think about the kind of medical care you would want to receive if you were seriously ill or facing a terminal diagnosis, and where you would want to be. Would you want what health care calls "life-prolonging care" (CPR, breathing machines, and anything else modern medicine has in its high-tech arsenal), "limited medical care" (which addresses treatable problems only), "comfort care" (aka palliative care, which focuses on people's comfort and ability to do as many of the things they love as possible), or some combination of all three?

2. Put your plan in writing. That plan is formalized in a document called an advance directive and is something you can create with the help of an attorney or on your own, using forms available for free online, from your doctor, or from your local hospital.

3. Give a copy of this document to each of your doctors and your loved ones, and use the occasion to initiate a conversation about your wishes.

4. Make sure your loved ones understand what you want and that you are entrusting them to speak for you if your condition or medication makes it impossible for you to speak for yourself. Designate one of them as your advocate.

COMMUNICATION BARRIERS AND ADVANCES

Chapter 2 covers the obstacles to productive communication that doctors and patients are facing today. These two sides continue to encounter major hurdles all the way up until the end of a patient's life. On the one hand, the patients and their families want hospital staff to really hear and empathize with them; to offer truthful, comprehensive, *early* information so that patients can make important choices about their treatment plan; and to be willing to carry out their wishes. On the other hand, staff have misconceptions about when end-of-life conversations should take place, lack the confidence to lead them, fail to include patients and families in decision making, and still find the subject of death just too difficult to tackle sometimes. A 2016 poll of US physicians found that "although 99 percent of the physicians feel end-of-life and advance-care-planning discussions are important, nearly half reported they do not know what to say and less than a third reported any prior training for these conversations."[3]

Enter several initiatives seeking to help patients and medical experts think and communicate about death—and living. The Conversation Project, started in 2010 by writers and other media members, clergy, and medical professionals, has a mission to "share the way we want to live through the end of our lives" and "communicate about the kind of care we want and don't want for ourselves."[4] It offers free, helpful conversation guides to start dialogues among caregivers, health care providers, family members, and others about what matters most to them. Additionally, death cafés—modeled after European *cafés philos* and *cafés scientifiques*—are increasingly popular gatherings designed for visitors to congregate and casually, confidentially discuss their mortality, "with a view to helping people make the most of their (finite) lives."[5]

On the provider side is the COMFORT model, a patient-centered communication framework that is training nurses to overcome conversational barriers with seriously ill patients. The acronym's seven principles—communication, orientation and opportunity, mindful communication, family, openings, relating, and team—are an important step toward bridging the divide that keeps getting in the way of the best possible care.[6] So are efforts by organizations like VitalTalk and the American Academy on Communication in Healthcare, both of which offer intensive in-person courses and online resources to health care professionals hoping for new ways to handle difficult communication tasks that arise in their work with end-of-life patients, and Harvard Medical School's Serious Illness Communication Guide and training program, which help physicians pursuing the same objective. The more public and professional interest we can generate in these kinds of ventures, the more everyone involved in talks about terminal illness, mortality, and end-of-life care will benefit.

HOW TO START THE CONVERSATION

So, how do you initiate a dialogue that could impact the rest of your life? The National Hospice and Palliative Care Organization has a booklet called "Conversations before the Crisis" that serves as an ideal starting point. It focuses on "conversation triggers" to make readers aware of the many possible paths to the start of the discussion. It also urges readers to begin to talk about the end of life while they are still healthy—hence the booklet's title. "Having these conversations before the crisis," the authors argue, "is not only much easier [but] much more valuable. . . . You will have made a significant contribution to your family, and you will discover important information for yourself."[7] Jennifer Temel, clinical director of thoracic oncology at Massachusetts General Hospital, adds that "one mistake we often make is only having these difficult conversations when something's going wrong. When someone's feeling terrible, and their family is very stressed that the patient is so sick, that's really not a time to have a calm and thoughtful conversation about prognosis and end-of-life care goals."[8]

People who embrace the early-intervention approach will find that "talk is the single most important thing that family and friends can do to prepare the end of life of someone they love. . . . Learning, insight, and love are possible to the last breath, and beyond. Talking about this time makes a rich ending more likely."[9]

The conversation triggers that the booklet mentions include:

• The death of a friend or colleague

• Newspaper articles about illness and funerals

• Movies

• Sermons

• Television talk shows, dramas, and comedies

• Financial planning

• Annual medical checkups

• Family occasions, such as baptisms, marriages, and (especially) funerals

• Magazines and books[10]

A family member wishing to initiate a conversation should be on the lookout for these cues and may be surprised by how frequently they pop up. Other factors to keep in mind are generational attitudes and sibling dynamics and potential conflicts (do all brothers and sisters in a family agree upon the best way to help their aging/ill parents?). Once the right opportunity presents itself, you'll be ready to start asking yourself and others the right questions to ensure a robust, meaningful exchange.

IMPORTANT QUESTIONS TO ASK

Harriet Warshaw, executive director of the Conversation Project, says that as you're preparing to open the avenues of communication with your loved ones and your doctor, you should "paint a picture of what matters most to you at the end of your life, because that will frame the kinds of treatment that you and your clinician will work on together."[11]

At the core of this conversation are questions such as:

- What matters most to me?

- What constitutes a joyful life to me?

- What is the meaning of comfort to me?

- Who do I want to be with at the end of my life? Where do I want to be? How do I want to be using my time?

- How and where do I want to receive treatment? Do I even want to receive treatment?

- What if things don't go well? How aggressive do I want my doctors and nurses to be?

- What if I can no longer speak for myself? Who do I want to speak for me?

- How should I pick my surrogate? Maybe it should not be the person who loves me the most—he or she may not be able to let me go if that is my choice.

- Have I shared my thoughts about these topics with my clinicians, my surrogate, and my family?

- Do I have an advance directive? Have I made copies of it, and do my loved ones and I know where they are?[12]

Thinking about these conversations thematically can also help to generate additional questions. In addition to the central question of what matters most to a patient, themes might include fears or worries (such as about pain) and how to express them, limits and trade-offs (where you "draw the line" in terms of your treatment preferences), and hospice care (which allows patients to receive care at home, have around-the-clock access to nursing professionals, and be assured of expert symptom management).[13]

No matter which specific questions resonate with you—or what other questions the list above inspires you to ask—the point is to ask them of yourself, your family, and your health care providers as early and as openly as you need to in order to ensure that your most important wishes are not only known but honored.

ADVANCE CARE PLANNING

Chapter 4 introduces the importance of advance care planning, which involves learning about the types of decisions that patients might need to make about the end of their life, considering those decisions ahead of time, and letting others—your family and your health care providers—know about your preferences. These preferences are then memorialized in an advance directive, a state-specific legal document that goes into effect only if the person becomes incapacitated and unable to speak on their own behalf, whether because of a disease or a severe injury. Despite the urgent need for all adults—even healthy ones—to have an advance directive in place, less than 50 percent of terminally ill patients have an advance directive, and more than 65 percent of doctors are not aware whether their patients have one.[14] No matter how old you are, an advance directive is essential because it makes others aware of what type of medical care you do or do not want to receive when you can no longer make your own decisions about such considerations as cardiopulmonary resuscitation (CPR); ventilator use; artificial nutrition (tube feeding) and artificial hydration; and comfort care (anything that can be done to soothe you or to relieve suffering, including managing shortness of breath; limiting medical tests; providing spiritual and emotional counseling; and taking medication for pain, anxiety, or general intestinal issues).

"Advance directive" is an umbrella term for various legal documents, which typically include a living will, a durable power of attorney, and a health care proxy. At some point, some medical professional, lawyer, or caregiver is going to ask you whether you have all these forms, so I want you to be familiar with the terminology before that conversation occurs.

- **Living will:** A living will alerts medical professionals and your family to the treatment you want to receive or refuse, and can describe under what conditions attempts to prolong your life should start or stop. Before a health care team uses a living will to guide medical decisions, two physicians must confirm that a patient is unable to make their own medical decisions and is in a medical condition that state law deems terminal illness or permanent unconsciousness. "Five Wishes" is an easy-to-complete living will that spells out in profound detail for the user's family and medical network not only what that person's medical needs are, but also what they want emotionally and spiritually. Its five categories are "The Person I Want to Make Health Care Decisions for Me When I Can't Make Them for Myself," "My Wish for the Kind of Medical Treatment I Want or Don't Want," "My Wish for How Comfortable I Want to Be," My Wish for How I Want People to Treat Me," and "My Wish for What I Want My Loved Ones to Know."[15]

• **Durable power of attorney:** A durable power of attorney for health care is a legal document in which you name someone (as well as a backup person, if you wish) as a proxy (agent) to make health care decisions for you if your physician declares you unable to do so. In that event, your proxy can speak on your behalf with your care team and make decisions according to the wishes or directions your durable power of attorney document specifies or, if your wishes are not specified, make decisions based on what they think you would want.

• **Health care proxy:** "Your health care proxy is like a designated driver who takes over decision-making when you are unable to advocate for yourself," says a Stanford Medicine blog post.[16] In this document, you designate the family member or trusted friend you want to play that role for you, and you give explicit directions about the details of the care you want. Always ask this person in advance whether they are willing to perform this role for you, and specify verbally, as well as in writing, what your health care wishes are.

Some states have an Advance Directive Registry where you can file your advance directive, so that you, your medical team, and your loved ones always know where a copy of it is. In addition, the AARP offers an online resource center that provides free advance-directive forms for every state, along with instructions for how to complete them and what to do with them.[17]

Also note that an advance directive is a *living document*—one that you can adjust as your situation changes because of new information or a change in your health. Whenever I've gone to advance-directive classes, the instructors emphasize that you can change these documents at any time—just because you put it in writing doesn't mean it's permanent. Even if you're already in the hospital, as long as you're still conscious, you can tell a loved one, "I've changed my mind about everything I said I wanted," and you can still update your legal documents to reflect your new instructions.

ADDITIONAL PAPERWORK

Documents you may also need to have on hand can provide critical information to help your medical team best serve your wishes.

Physician Orders for Life-Sustaining Treatment (POLST) Form

A POLST form also helps describe a person's health care wishes, but it is not an advance directive. Instead, it is a set of specific medical orders that describe the person's wishes in an emergency: whether to use CPR, whether to go to a hospital, whether to be put on a breathing machine, and so forth. A seriously ill person can complete the form and ask a qualified member of their health care team to sign it. Emergency personnel—that is, paramedics and emergency medical technicians—*cannot* use an advance directive, but they *can* use a POLST form. Without a POLST form, these personnel must perform every possible measure to keep the patient alive.[18]

Organ and Tissue Donation Registration

If you are interested in donating your organs and tissues upon your death, donor registries, such as Donate Life and your state's Department of Motor Vehicles, make offering your consent convenient and provide an electronic record of your decision. When you register, you can save the lives of up to eight people (through organ donation) and seventy-five people (through tissue donation) awaiting heart, lung, kidney, liver, pancreas, and other transplants.[19]

Do Not Resuscitate (DNR) Order

Resuscitation means that medical staff will try to restart your heart and breathing using methods such as CPR (cardiopulmonary resuscitation) and AED (automated external defibrillator). In some cases, they may also use life-sustaining devices, such as breathing machines. The primary reason signing a DNR order is important is that if you do not speak up for yourself and specify what you want—and if you do not have a patient advocate who can back you up—the default treatment that you're going to get is risky. If you are in a state of profound distress or your body shuts down, your medical team is going to perform CPR on you. And lest you think CPR is a cure-all and that you'll be magically alive, the same way you were before, you should know that only 10.6 percent of patients who receive CPR following cardiac arrest recover enough to be discharged from the hospital.[20] More often than not, the following scenario is likely: A woman in her seventies or eighties who does not have an advance directive and who is very ill begins to have difficulty breathing, and her heart stops. When the EMTs do CPR on her, they break her ribs. Now, in addition to her preexisting conditions, even though she can technically breathe again, she has broken ribs that cause her constant pain. On top of that, she might get pneumonia—or she doesn't wake up at all because she's brain-dead from the CPR. Even entering a hospital puts patients at risk. They can get MRSA. They can get a urinary tract infection. They don't want to be there, and they need to get out as quickly as possible so that they can be in a more sanitary environment, but how are they going to do that when the interventions that their medical team has performed have only guaranteed them an even longer stay? In the worst-case scenarios, a 2017 *New York Times* article revealed, even patients who have created an advance directive, a POLST form or a Medical Orders for Life-Sustaining Treatment (MOLST) form, have had doctors violate their explicit directions and perform unwanted lifesaving measures.[21]

These grave scenarios start with the fact that when some-one goes to a hospital, they have so many people taking care of them. In addition, the communication lines in the hospital are sometimes so poor that certain members of the care team don't even know the patient has a DNR in the first place because there's not a consistent chain of communication among all the medical teams who are helping this patient. So, not only does a patient need to have the critical end-of-life conversations with their family and their health care provider and have all their paper-work in order, but, in a perfect world, their care team would find a way to distribute the patient's wishes to the entire group, so that every person who comes in and takes care of the patient at any point in the day sees the necessary documents and knows what the patient wants should an emergency arise. No matter how many years a doctor has spent in school and practicing medicine, no matter how many times they've been instructed to save their patients' lives, they need to work for the patient, not for the patient's disease. They need to remember that a patient is a person who has specific rights, and they need to honor their wishes. If the patient wants to stay alive as long as possible, no matter what it takes, that's one thing. But if they don't want to suffer anymore, they need to have that option available to them when they want it, no questions asked. That's what advance care planning is all about.

WHAT NEXT?

Once you have all your affairs in order, the ideal next step is to tell your whole family and any other important friends or care-givers about the decisions you've made, and ideally to make sure that everyone is on the same page. When my mother died, I was her health care proxy, and I was very cognizant that I wanted her experience to be peaceful. I didn't want anyone hysterical around her. When I saw that she was dying, my father, my brothers, and I sang some of her favorite songs together until she stopped breathing. After she died, my father said to me, "That's how I want to go too." One of my brothers and I had a disagreement over our dad's DNR order—he was questioning me about it—but my father had already made up his mind. He had a DNR bracelet, and the local hospital had a record of the order. This is just one of countless examples of situations in which the patient needs to figure out their wishes and decide whom they really trust to carry them out. Just because you have it in writing doesn't mean you might not get some resistance from other family members who are not the patient's health care proxy, but once it's written down, no one besides the patient can change the plan. You've simply got to honor your loved one and find a way to accept their decisions.

AMY BERMAN

I introduced you to Amy Berman in chapter 1. She is the ultimate example of how life-changing the decision to consult a palliative care specialist—and doing so *early*—can be for a terminally ill patient. If Berman had accepted her original oncologist's recommendations and started with radiation, chemotherapy, and a mastectomy right after she was diagnosed, she would most likely be dead already and would have suffered profoundly before then. Instead, she sought a second opinion, received a one-time dose of radiation, and has continued to work and travel since her diagnosis, despite the fact that she continues to have cancer. This woman did everything right in terms of advocating for herself, and those actions have led her to a greatly improved quality of life.

Berman has said of her experience, "The advance care planning conversations I have had with my health care team have been lifesaving since my diagnosis. I use the word 'lifesaving' advisedly because that is what these conversations are truly about. When done well, they can shape care in ways that give people with serious illness a chance at getting the best life possible. . . . Quality of life is more important to me than quantity of days, if they are miserable days."[22]

Berman is just one of the many examples of the value of speaking up and taking a stand for one's body, mind, and spirit. Doing so can literally save a person's life. I give her tremendous credit for being so courageous. To take such matters into your own hands, you really have to know not just what you don't want—surgery, chemo, radiation—but also what you *do* want. And when no one has the answer about what the outcome will be in lieu of the standard treatment, the gamble is even greater. I don't even know what I would do if David came back and our family was in the same scenario again. But for Amy Berman, things worked out better in the end. So many people out there are in similar situations now that if this book can find them and empower them to use their voices in the same way, I will have done the job I set out to do by writing it.

FINAL THOUGHTS

The American way of life is very pragmatic in general. We tend to set goals and then rush toward them, and often work long hours, sometimes seven days per week. Not surprisingly, then, when someone finds out they have a serious illness, they often end up being so busy fighting it that they forget they also need to live a little along the way. They rush to kill the disease, to beat it, to be winners. It's wonderful if things work out that way eventually. But in the meantime, while all the hard stuff is happening, you're still alive and you need to take advantage of it.

To facilitate your pursuit of well-being, deal with all the logistical tasks this chapter mentions, and do it now, so that you don't have to tackle them later and so that you can live a full and rich life. Have the difficult conversations with your family and your health care team. Get all your paperwork squared away. Then, when the time comes that you do need medical intervention, all of your wishes are documented, everybody is aware of them, and you can rest assured that you've done everything you can do to advocate for yourself. In doing so, you will clear space for yourself to slow down, to smell the proverbial roses, to really enjoy however much time you have left—whether that's weeks, months, or decades.

Amy Berman says, "Perhaps the most troubling issue palliative care faces is the public misperception that palliative care means giving up. This couldn't be further from the truth."[23] Rather, palliative care, which includes the steps outlined in this chapter, is a gateway to self-empowerment, one that allows people to get down to the business of not simply existing but really living.

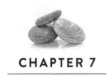

CHAPTER 7

Spirituality and Well-Being

CARE OF THE SPIRIT MATTERS TOO

It isn't until you come to a spiritual understanding of who
you are—not necessarily a religious feeling, but deep down,
the spirit within—that you can begin to take control.

—OPRAH WINFREY, TALK SHOW HOST, TELEVISION PRODUCER,
ACTRESS, AUTHOR, AND PHILANTHROPIST

The diagnosis of a serious or life-threatening condition brings into sharp focus what is truly important to you. You may find yourself examining how you've lived your life up to this point and wondering about its purpose. Has it been meaningful to you? To others? It is not unusual for a sense of loss to set in— loss of illusions, loss of self, loss of hope. In palliative care, this state of mind is referred to as spiritual distress. It taps into the idea that pain isn't just physical—it is also psychological, social, cultural, and spiritual, and it encompasses the whole person.

After David's stem cell transplant, when his favorite physician agreed to talk to him about the big life questions David had been pondering, our son finally had the conversation he needed to feel seen and whole. The American College of Physicians has noted that medical doctors "have the obligation to attend to all dimensions of the patient's illness experience—the psychosocial, spiritual, and existential suffering, as well as physical pain."[1] Yet spiritual suffering is an aspect of illness that modern American medicine ignores. In contrast, palliative care has always recognized that attending to a person's spirituality is an essential element of improving quality of life, because serious physical distress is accompanied by spiritual distress. We have Dame Cicely Saunders, the founder of hospice, to thank for this valuable understanding. Saunders "dedicated her life to the care of dying patients by attending to the 'total pain' of the patient, a term she described as encompassing spiritual distress, as well as psychosocial and physical distress. Her model . . . emphasizes the totality of a patient's experience in the context of their illness and/or dying."[2]

As Christina Puchalski, MD, director of the George Washington Institute for Spirituality and Health at George Washington University School of Medicine and Health Sciences in Washington, DC, and author of *Making Health Care Whole: Integrating Spirituality into Patient Care*, explains, "Spiritual care is not about fixing and resolving spiritual distress with a pill. It is instead the recognition that people can find healing within themselves, even in the midst of dying. . . . Spiritual care emphasizes whole health even in the midst of serious disease and dying. The focus is shifted from disease to health and well-being. Spiritual care, therefore, is, at its root, honoring the dignity of each person and providing care that is based in compassion."[3]

David had not received compassionate support from his health care team, and as a result he suffered from a lack of attentiveness to who he was as a person. Integrating palliative care into mainstream, modern American medicine presents a different picture, one in which the spiritual needs of patients and families are as important as any other aspect of care.

SPIRITUALITY AND RELIGION

Let's begin by exploring the key differences between religion and spirituality. The former is a set of institutionalized beliefs and practices, often based on the teachings of a historical figure, such as Jesus Christ or the Buddha. The latter is typically a more abstract, more individualized relationship between a person and the idea of something "bigger" than they are. My opinion is that all religion is spiritual on some level, but not all spiritual feelings and thoughts are religious. Religion has a long history, dating back to ancient times, of being used to guide—and sometimes control—various populations. Spirituality, meanwhile, is much broader and more abstract and has not gotten the full attention that it deserves. In the case of palliative care, it emphasizes finding healing from within, identifying with a compassionate presence, and eventually finding peace and well-being within this very difficult encounter with pain and suffering. Or, as Puchalski explains it, "Spirituality is the aspect of humanity that refers to the way individuals seek and express meaning and purposes and the way they experience their connectedness to the moment, to self, to others, to nature, and to the significant or sacred."[4]

A 2020 Fetzer Institute study, "What Does Spirituality Mean to Us?," sought to better understand spirituality in the United States today by asking people about how they understand and experience spirituality for themselves and how their spirituality relates to the way they engage with others and their community. This group included people inside and outside religious institutions, those who considered themselves spiritual, and those who did not. The Fetzer project resonated with me because it demonstrated that spirituality is a universal concept and does not pigeonhole people in one group, as religion does. It brings people together, rather than creating barriers. Other key revelations included the following:

- **Spirituality is a shared human experience:** Most people consider themselves spiritual to some extent, and they say that spirituality is important in their lives. For many, spirituality also represents the type of person they want to be: people are becoming more spiritual over their own lives, see being spiritual as an aspiration to strive for, and describe spiritual people in positive terms.

• **Spirituality is about depth and nuance:** Spiritual identity—that is, calling oneself spiritual—is only one of many measures of what it means to live a spiritual life. People identify a wide range of encounters and activities as spiritual, and they are regularly engaging in them or seeking them out both within and outside religious institutions.

• **Spirituality is connected with an engaged civic life:** People who identify as highly spiritual are more likely to say it is important to make a difference in their communities and contribute to greater good in the world. They are also more likely to be politically engaged.

• **Spirituality broadens perspectives:** People vary in terms of how much they connect with their own spirituality and how they interact with the world. In focus-group conversations about this relationship, participants who identified as having a spiritually driven outer life often opened others' eyes to a connection between their own spirituality and the actions they take.[5]

Finally, the study highlighted the fact that not all religious or spiritual people believe in some sort of higher power, as some "react against the word 'God,' but some find that word central to their faith. Some find that 'higher power' does not speak to the kind of present, loving, and all-knowing being that they envision. For many, thinking of the divine as 'universal energy' is perfect; for others it is not adequately personal." Regardless of how anyone defines it, spiritual experiences like these "have been shown to fuel people's faith, propel them to act in the world in loving ways, and influence how people give of themselves to others."[6] Another study found that spirituality and religiosity are "correlated with reduced morbidity and mortality, better physical and mental health, healthier lifestyles, fewer required health services, improved coping skills, enhanced well-being, reduced stress, and illness prevention."[7]

If spiritual bliss can be interpreted as "love from God, selfless love from others, transcendent presence through awe of creation, and gratitude for life," among other responses, imagine, then, what the opposite—spiritual distress—feels like. I first heard Puchalski discuss the concept in 2019, during a talk she gave at the Kanarek Center for Palliative Care at Fairfield University. When people asked her about the most common signs of spiritual distress, she said, "There's depression. There's anger. There are personality changes. There's belligerence." These behaviors were exactly what David exhibited when he was in strict isolation following his stem cell transplant, yet the health care professionals treating him at the time never gave his personality change a name; instead, they just kept saying that they saw similar responses in a lot of children who were having transplants. My gut reaction when I started to notice David's changes was to recall my readings of Elisabeth Kübler-Ross, who talks a lot about existential issues, and I just had a hunch that he had questions about his mortality. But as soon as I heard Puchalski's lecture, I knew that what David had gone through wasn't just an existential crisis—she was the one who gave the most accurate name to what I had witnessed in my child: spiritual distress.

People who are in the midst of spiritual distress generally do not know to call it that. They might just feel worthless; they might be losing weight; they might be anxious, depressed, angry, or even self-blaming. I'll never forget when David relapsed. We were at the doctor's office, and when I told him his cancer had come back, he asked me, "Why me? What did I do wrong?" Joe and I asked the same questions when David was first diagnosed—we kept asking his doctor if there was anything that we could have done to prevent his cancer, or if we had caused it some way, even if genetically. She was a typical, stoic New Englander and a strict Catholic, but she just looked at us and said, "Mr. and Mrs. Kanarek, this falls under the title 'Shit Happens.'" It was an excellent answer. David's cancer just happened to us; we didn't do anything wrong. And it might not happen to you, but it could happen to the person standing right next to you. It's just one of those senseless things in life.

Because of the gravity of a terminal diagnosis and all the doubt it raises, patients themselves rarely recognize the changes they undergo as a result. Their family members are usually the ones who have to acknowledge the negative transformation that they've witnessed in their loved one and say, "You may not be able to recognize it, but you are in spiritual distress and you need to get help." In David's case, it was up to me to say to his doctors, "This is not my son."

"Spiritual distress" resonated so strongly with me as a description for what David was going through that soon after that lecture I wrote an essay about my epiphany, entitled "Spiritual Distress Manifested in a Teenager after a Stem Cell Transplant," for the *Journal of Pain and Symptom Management*.[8] All the questions David had been seeking answers to—"Why me?" "What did I do to deserve this?" "Where is God?" "Where am I in all this?"—took a severe toll on him. Just imagine what it's like when you know that you have a life-threatening condition and you're in isolation or in a private hospital room, with zero access to the outside world and few to no visitors. And among the family members and friends and anyone else who does visit, none of them has the same problem. None of them is worried they're not going to come out of this. When you're in that situation, you stop knowing what normal is. Your mind starts playing games with you.

If someone is in spiritual distress, they have to be able to express it to somebody so that it doesn't fester. Once they begin externalizing it, their ability to resist the physical symptoms of their illness improves because they don't have to bear such a heavy emotional burden on their own. David finally got the relief he sought when someone took the time to talk to him at length about what he was feeling—someone compassionate, someone trustworthy, someone who could just sit with him in that state and really listen to whatever he had to get off his chest. That's what spiritual care is all about. It's not about trying to find a solution to the patient's woes, because chances are that after the patient goes through an experience with a certified palliative care professional, they will find the solution from within. They will finally understand what their feelings are about and why they have them.

I remember when a financial-planner friend of mine once contacted me to say that he was meeting with a family who had just lost a child in an accident. He was terrified about what his role was going to be, so he called me and asked, "What should I do?"

I said, "Honestly, sit there and listen and offer them tissues. Lean forward. Just really take in their information. Do not give advice—just listen." He was with them for an hour, doing just that, and when he left, they said, "We cannot tell you how much you've helped us." Even if he barely spoke during the meeting, they felt entirely supported by the way he communicated with them. If you find yourself in the same position, don't bring your personal issues into the situation; just listen. It's a real art form. As Puchalski says, "The clinician who listens intentionally and with full presence creates an environment of trust, where the patient . . . can share what is of deep concern." This kind of deep interaction can allow the patient "to find a way to cope with suffering . . . to find peace and well-being."[9]

We know that for seriously ill patients, spiritual support via palliative care can provide a better quality of life, a greater ability to cope with a terminal diagnosis, and greater psychosocial function. Whether you are formally religious or broadly spiritual, the manifestation of these benefits depends on how well your health care provider does at making you feel heard and understood. For example, if you are Muslim or Jewish, you may need to observe specific cultural considerations during a hospitalization, related to periods of rest, dietary laws, times for prayer, modesty guidelines, and even rules about eye contact. Some hospitals are already honoring such preferences while treating religiously observant patients, but if your facility does not initiate a conversation with you about your needs, you should never hesitate to bring them up on your own.

While some patients derive tangible advantages from access to a religious leader, such as a rabbi or a chaplain, during their illness, others need professionals who have expertise in the realm of spirituality at large. Even if you don't follow an institutionalized religion, an illness can bring up your own spiritual beliefs and experiences from the past, as well as a wide range of questions, thoughts, and feelings, including questions about the deeper meaning of your life or your place in the universe, regrets you may have about your past or decisions you have made, what is important to you now, what your main fears and sources of strength are, and what role your family and friends have in your illness. Palliative care must address these crucial existential and spiritual questions and help to ease the way for patients who are undergoing such an intense period of inquiry.

PROVIDING SPIRITUAL SUPPORT FOR FAMILY AND FRIENDS

Although spiritual care requires professional guidance, we know from chapter 6 that palliative care involves a patient's entire family-and-friends network. If you are among the people supporting someone with a serious illness, you can be instrumental in bolstering their sense of spiritual well-being. The National Hospice and Palliative Care Organization has the following advice for patients' loved ones:

- **Be aware of the nature of spiritual pain and suffering:**
  Understand that the patient may be questioning the overall
  meaning of life and whether they have made a positive
  impact with their own; may be feeling guilty about things
  they have done or blaming others for things that have
  happened to them; may be questioning their long-held
  religious beliefs; and may be feeling alienated from their
  faith community.

- **Be present:** Realize that a caring presence and the ability
  to listen is sometimes the best gift you can give your loved
  one.

- **Ask open, supportive questions:** Gently invite your loved
  one to have a conversation about spiritual matters; you
  can open the discussion by saying something like, "I was
  wondering if you might want to talk to me about how your
  illness is affecting you spiritually."

- **Listen with an open heart:** Listen carefully and without
  judgment to whatever your loved one wants to share, and
  be open to any emotions that arise. The expression of feelings is an integral part of the search for spiritual healing.

- **Offer compassionate support:** Focus on the other person,
  not on your experience; express your support and love;
  be sincere.

- **Use spiritual resources and rituals as appropriate:**
  Request the patient's permission first; then, if you receive
  it, ask if the person has a favorite prayer, religious reading,
  or hymn that you could enjoy together.

- **Remember that you are not in this alone:** Encourage the
  involvement of clergy, chaplains, or other spiritual leaders
  who have expertise in spiritual care; know your own comfort zone and boundaries in this arena.[10]

Talking about illness and end-of-life care can be difficult and emotional for friends and family members of patients. The urge to skirt the issues and say, "Don't talk like that," "Don't lose hope," or "Stay positive," when someone brings up death and dying is sometimes powerful. However, try to keep in mind that this fear can present a hindrance for your loved ones when they are already struggling with profound questions about the meaning of life. The best gift you can give them is to do your "emotional homework" and be brave enough to confront head-on the topics that they want to address in order to have a smooth and peaceful journey in whatever time they have remaining.

THE PALLIATIVE CARE "DREAM TEAM"

When we first noticed David's personality begin to change when he was in isolation after his transplant, we brought in a psychiatrist—who did *not* specialize in palliative care—to try to help him. But the man simply started treating David with Freudian strategies that involved discussing potential issues with me, and the whole undertaking was fruitless. Not only was David *not* struggling with the mother-son relationship, he wasn't looking for someone to psychoanalyze him using a one-size-fits-all approach. He just needed someone who could listen intently and carefully, who was trained to ask some leading questions that would ultimately empower him to answer his own questions, and who could validate what he was feeling. That's why it is so important that a palliative care designation exists in the medical field—so that patients with life-threatening diseases have access to certified experts who know the right way to talk to people in distress, rather than just feeding the patients falsely optimistic stories when they're eager to grab on to any shred of hope. People with serious illnesses are extremely vulnerable and impressionable. When pseudo-professionals—service providers who are not fully educated or who have not reached a certain skill level—are incorporated into a care team, they are more likely to promote their personal agenda, take patients' money, and do more damage than good. Only if your primary doctor is really advocating for someone and knows their training background and if your whole team is on the same page should you feel confident about engaging that person's services.

Some health care providers don't even attempt to acknowledge when a patient is under unusual duress. For instance, when Joe and I commented to David's physicians on the changes we were observing in our son, they just kept telling us, "This is normal." We had to stand our ground to have any chance of being heard. We said, "Okay. If it's normal, if it happens to everybody, does that mean we just accept it as is?" That's when we convinced David's doctor to go in and see David and spend that three-hour period with him. If a person breaks his leg, he can't walk. *That's* normal. But unless somebody comes and sets the leg and puts it in a cast, the person will never walk again. David needed the equivalent of a cast for his psyche.

Ideally, anyone who helps a seriously ill patient will have a high-level understanding of spirituality, which ties in with the whole-person care for which I've advocated throughout this book. The desire for spiritual guidance among patients is certainly strong: One study showed that between 50 and 95 percent of cancer patients, for one, view religion and/or spirituality as personally important to them, and also that most of those patients feel as if the medical community supports their spiritual needs only minimally or not at all.[11] Another, a survey of 921 patients, revealed that the majority believed information about their spiritual beliefs would affect physicians' ability to encourage realistic hope (67 percent), give medical advice (66 percent), and change medical treatment (62 percent).[12]

If a patient is thinking, *My life is over*, that represents a profound state of spiritual distress. In a perfect world, whoever is the recipient of that patient's existential questions would have the tools to examine the patient's psyche and ask a series of specific questions designed to inspire the patient to open up. If that doesn't work, the health care provider should next say, "I might not be the right person to help to ease your suffering, but I'm going to immediately take action and direct you to someone who can." As the Palliative Care Network of Wisconsin notes,

> Spiritual care generalists, nurses, social workers, physicians, and other [interdisciplinary team] clinicians have the responsibility to screen for spiritual distress and spiritual needs as part of the consultation or history and physical process. . . . This includes listening for phrases [that] may indicate a need for spiritual support, such as: "Why is this happening to me?," "What God would allow this?," "I still have things to do in my life!," or "I've lost touch with my faith leader since I've been in the hospital. . . ." Clinicians should refer to a chaplain if unmet spiritual needs and/or spiritual distress are suspected.[13]

Chaplains trained in palliative care both provide spiritual and religious support to patients and family members and can also support their coworkers in hospital settings. In addition, says the Joint Commission, which accredits health care organizations and programs across the United States, "When health care providers feel cared for, they are rejuvenated and can provide better care to their patients and family members." In addition, the Joint Commission "requires health care leaders to make support systems available to staff who have been involved in an adverse or sentinel event through the Leadership Standard, and chaplains can play a vital part of that support system."[14]

Unfortunately, despite the American College of Physicians' exhortation to medical doctors to attend to all dimensions of the patient's illness experience, the contrast between what doctors would ideally do and the support they actually offer continues to be stark. Although more than 80 percent of US medical schools offer spiritual training courses, they are elective, not mandatory, and formal systems of communication between physicians and chaplains in hospitals are limited.[15] Thus, because doctors and nurses are not trained to be comfortable with the subject of spiritual distress, even if they encounter patients requesting guidance, they lack either the skill set or the time to help. Physicians are also not attending to their patients' whole selves because they are too focused on pain management and diagnosis and following a prescribed course of treatment—too busy trying to heal physical and psychosocial issues to focus on the more abstract ones or to ask themselves, "Can we also do anything about the *other* issues this patient is enduring?" When they sit there and simply listen to a patient in spiritual distress, they feel as if they're "not doing anything," rather than realizing that they're actually making a tremendous impact. Puchalski says it's all about "recognizing that conversations are important in clinical care and not just end-of-life care. Every single visit I have with a patient includes a conversation about spirituality, about what's important to them. Every time we come to a crossroads that requires a decision, I want to know: 'Where are you today, what's important to you, what gives your life meaning and value, and how does this affect your decisions?'"[16]

A full complement of palliative care professionals—a patient's "dream team"—comprises a wide range of roles, including doctors, nurses, and palliative medicine/pain specialists; psychiatrists, psychologists, and social workers; spiritual counselors, grief counselors, and religious leaders; physical therapists and massage therapists; dieticians; and even attorneys. These people would all share goals about improving their patients' quality of life and would include specialists who were certified in palliative care, whenever possible. No matter what a provider's specific job title is, palliative care–specific training is almost always available to them. The College of Pastoral Supervision and Psychotherapy, for example, offers training and accreditation for chaplains, pastoral supervisors, and pastoral psychotherapists. The National Association of Social Workers and the National Hospice and Palliative Care Organization award palliative care certification to qualified social workers. A specialty palliative care certification has been available to nurses since 1994 through the Hospice and Palliative Care Credentialing Center. And the American Board of Medical Specialties and American Osteopathic Association administer a specialty examination for palliative medicine physicians.[17]

In addition, a number of spiritual assessment tools are helping palliative care providers to know the right questions to ask patients who are suffering from spiritual distress. The first is the HOPE spiritual assessment, which can be used to assess the spiritual needs of the ill. The second is the FICA, the letters of which stand for *faith*, *importance and influence*, *community*, and *address*, and which Puchalski intended to be part of a patient's regular screening during an annual exam or initial intake appointment. The third tool is the SPIRIT assessment, which explores questions related to personal belief systems, religious communities, and religious practices and the implications of those factors for medical care and terminal-event planning. Any provider can use these frameworks to gain more insight into a patient's spiritual needs.[18]

Some patients want people to vent to, and others want more active counseling from specialists who can ask them deeper, more targeted questions and help them try to make sense of what they're going through. Either way, access to a wide variety of such experts should be a prerequisite for any successful palliative care program, and all of those care providers need to be prepared to address the issues that patients bring up, even when that means not so much talking to them as listening while they unburden themselves of all their fears, all their concerns, all the questions that they need answered.

FOSTERING EXISTENTIAL AND
SPIRITUAL STRENGTHS

A prominent aspect of the spiritual care equation is helping patients who are experiencing spiritual distress to understand that what they think of as normal life is going to look very different from now on, and that that's okay. While the new normal is not the same as the old normal, it can be a very reasonable standard of life. Effective spiritual care teaches patients to deal with negative thought patterns, so that instead of thinking, for example, *If I can't get back to running, my life will be over*, they begin realizing, *I might not be able to get back to running, but I have lots of other hobbies that I can still enjoy, and I may even pick up some new ones*. Some things may be taken away from you, but other good things will show up to take their place.

My daughter, Sarah, who works as an occupational therapist at Memorial Sloan Kettering, has a lot of patients who are debilitated after their treatments. Because she has established a rapport with them, she has found that people will start asking her questions about their future, including "Am I going to be able to return to normal?" The fact is, focusing on trying to get back to where you were before you got sick is counterproductive at times. What you should be setting your sights on instead— and here's where a palliative care team of spiritually minded experts can have a major impact—is identifying what is important to you and then working with your team to achieve those objectives. With the right experiences and the right guidance, patients who have given up hope can find their zest for life again. One way to understand spiritual palliative care, says a team of researchers who synthesized extensive studies on the topic in 2020, "is as an approach that can contribute to quality of life by identifying and supporting existential or spiritual strengths of patients," which fall into five primary categories: meaning, connection, personal agency, faith, and hope.[19] The researchers explain that these groups "can be visualized as separate, yet interlinked, strengthening each other. Much like the blades of a propeller." They propose that this framework raises "*awareness* that there are specific approaches that can lead to patient experiences of existential or spiritual strength, and that these ways are important from a distress-reducing perspective, and from a view-point of (final) human flourishing. . . . The existential or spiritual is often found in everyday, simple things, and is mostly not situated in an otherworldly dimension out *there*, but in an essential dimension right *here*." The propeller framework is a useful way for palliative care professionals to better coordinate their patient care and stimulate patients' perceptions of the positive aspects of their existence, even during illness.[20]

One of my favorite metaphors about life is that it's like a balloon: you squeeze in one place, and it bulges somewhere else. A specialist working with patients who lose a leg, for example, will teach them to deal with the loss by helping them to understand how to squeeze their own proverbial balloon and thus overemphasize other abilities they still possess. Whether you're doing occupational or physical therapy, trying out any of the alternative therapies I touched on in chapter 5, or actively seeking to foster your spiritual strengths, the path to inner equilibrium and peace is in front of you. At some point, something *will* click within you and brighten you up. It's just a question of redirecting your energy. Remember Amy Berman from chapter 1? The one thing she was really adamant about following her cancer diagnosis was that she didn't want to be debilitated by chemotherapy. She was determined to continue working and traveling. Those were the things she needed to do to find the meaning that Viktor Frankl accentuates in his book *Man's Search for Meaning*. Like Berman, even if you find yourself in the most difficult circumstances of your life so far, you have to discover within yourself a way to move forward. In order to find the light, you sometimes have to get down into a ditch. That's where you access the inner strength to go forward. As Frankl says, "When we are no longer able to change a situation, we are challenged to change ourselves" and "Everything can be taken from a man but one thing: the last of the human freedoms—to choose one's attitude in any given set of circumstances, to choose one's own way."[21]

THE NEED FOR HOPE

In May 2019, Rabbi Mark Golub, founder and host of the Jewish Broadcasting Service, interviewed me about palliative care, my Jewish background, my nursing background, and my experience with David's illness. At one point, he asked me, "Right after the diagnosis, did you give up hope?" I remember being struck by that. I told him—and he appeared quite surprised by my response—"We had hope until the moment David died!"[22] To me, hope—especially when you're dealing with an ill child—is what keeps you going. Joe and I could not allow ourselves to think that David's illness was going to end the way it did, because that mindset would have paralyzed us. So all we focused on was trying to make things better for him, trying to free him from his own suffering, and never giving up. And David absorbed all that hope we were holding on to. Even when he was two years old, if he fell and hurt himself, the first thing he did was to look at us, his parents. We never flinched, so he never cried when he fell. We modeled that same behavior for him throughout his diagnosis and treatment, right up until his death.

Hope is part of everybody's life before they experience a serious illness or injury. It's with us all the time, even if we're not thinking about it. But then everything changes with a diagnosis. However, if you're committed to achieving quality of life and preserving what matters with you day-to-day, hope continues to be equally important, if not more so.

Cynthia Cramer, a clinical administrative supervisor at Tampa General Hospital and a palliative care resource nurse, explains that

> hope is a very fluid thing. It changes depending on where you are on the trajectory of life. For newly diagnosed patients . . . , the hope is for a cure. With more advanced [illnesses], the hope may be for control. . . . And if control is not a possibility, there is always hope for time. Time to finish business, to tell someone "I'm sorry," to leave a legacy, to experience something special like a graduation or a marriage, or maybe even time for that "magic drug" to be invented. . . . And finally, there is hope for a "good death."
> . . . Patients are where they want to be, as comfortable as possible, doing what they want to do, surrounded by the people they love, with their symptoms well managed and their goals accomplished.[23]

If we revisit the propeller framework we explored earlier in this chapter, you'll recall that hope is one of the five "blades" that represent spiritual or existential strength. The authors of this study observed that four pursuits have the potential to enhance hope: (1) setting special targets (such as goals to attend particular events or reach certain personal benchmarks); (2) imagining alternate outcomes (such as fantasizing about a cure for an incurable illness or about continuing to be a presence in loved ones' lives after death); (3) building a collection of objects and mementos, such as photographs, writings, and music; and (4) extending wishes for loved ones' future through legacy documents and conversations.[24] The key takeaway here is that hope may change shape and appear in all kinds of different forms, but it's never out of reach. It's up to patients, and their families, friends, and caregivers, to harness it and keep it alive.

FINAL THOUGHTS

Spirituality in palliative care has not received the attention it deserves, partly because of confusion about what spirituality encompasses in the first place. Is it religious, or is it existential? The answer depends on an individual's particular perspective, but generally, while spirituality is not necessarily religious in nature, religion is one element of spirituality.

Spirituality becomes important to patients as they approach their own death, and spiritual well-being makes the changes in their quality of life less onerous and makes them more resilient as they cope with a terminal illness. Spiritual care is thus not about fixing a problem but rather about healing from within. This is where the provider-patient relationship becomes critical. The conversations that occur between the two parties do not happen easily or quickly; they are intimate and protracted, with the goal of allowing the patient to be heard on many levels. That acknowledgment alone can have a profoundly healing effect, as David demonstrated during his illness.

Nurses and doctors encounter many patients who ask for guidance about their spiritual plight. They may be experiencing anger, anxiety, or depression; feeling bewildered about their diagnosis; and unable to process their inner turmoil. Health care providers who are not trained to deal with spiritual issues must refer the patient to a palliative care social worker, psychologist, or chaplain—someone who can help the ill person give voice to and make sense of what they are enduring. Patient rights include religious and spiritual rights, and we must strive to hold health care facilities and their staff accountable for honoring these rights as we advance the cause of palliative care, and for taking an interprofessional approach that targets a patient's body, mind, and spirit equally. In the meantime, as we pursue these goals, patients must continue to be their own best advocates and specifically request a palliative care–certified social worker, chaplain, or psychologist to attend to them when they need assistance in sorting out and legitimizing their feelings. Spiritual distress is not limited to patients. It affects their families, their caregivers, and other health professionals alike—everybody who's involved with the patient's diagnosis and treatment—and often prompts all these groups to engage in intense self-reflection. Joe and I came face-to-face with profound spiritual distress while David was still alive and continue to struggle with it now, more than two decades after his death. But through a variety of support channels, through sharing our family's journey through his illness, and through discovering books like Frankl's *Man's Search for Meaning*, we have found our own ways to accept our circumstances. In life-and-death situations, the questions that arise—about mortality, about meaning, about what we've done and who we are—are too important to ignore. Everyone deserves the opportunity to find the answers they seek.

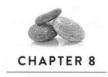

CHAPTER 8

Grief

TAPPING INTO RESTORATIVE SOURCES AFTER GOODBYE

*You will not "get over" the loss of a loved one; you will
learn to live with it. You will heal and you will rebuild
yourself around the loss you have suffered. You will be
whole again but you will never be the same. Nor should
you be the same, nor would you want to.*

—ELISABETH KÜBLER-ROSS, MD (1926–2004), PSYCHIATRIST
AND PIONEER IN NEAR-DEATH STUDIES

It is said that grief is the price we pay for love. Our love for David
was boundless; when he died, our grief blocked out the sun.
Often it even felt like a huge wave that kept crashing over us. It
would come out of nowhere and leave us inconsolable, sometimes in public. We had no control over it. We were exhausted
emotionally and physically. Nothing made sense; mundane
events like grocery shopping somehow angered me. I agonized
about how David might have felt at the end and found it impossible not to replay over and over again some of the most trying
moments during his last hospitalization. I wondered if I would
ever feel "normal" again.

For the first two or three years after David's death, I experienced brain fog—also called griever's fog, widow's fog, or trauma
fog—a common condition that occurs after a significant loss or
traumatic experience. When a person experiences such a loss,
the resulting devastation triggers their pituitary gland to release
adrenocorticotrophin (ACTH). The ACTH then sends a signal to

the adrenal glands to release cortisol, a stress hormone. The person's body remains flooded with cortisol for several months, or even longer.[1] For me, brain fog manifested itself in the form of long-term memory loss and crippling fatigue. There are several periods of time after David's death that I still cannot remember. For example, I went to Norway to visit a friend. I met one of her neighbors and invited her to visit us in London. When I went back to Norway several years later, I bumped into the neighbor and invited her to London again. She reminded me that she had already visited. I said, "I completely forgot!" and to this day, I have no memory of her coming to see me. People would say, "Oh, don't you remember I told you such-and-such?" or, "I told you that!" I would have to say, "I'm sorry. There's a whole part of my brain that just isn't remembering certain things right now." They were mostly accepting, but at times I thought I might even have early-onset Alzheimer's. Today, I know that the severe lapse I experienced is a neurological by-product of profound trauma and grief. I also know that people who have a friend or relative experiencing the loss of a loved one should be made aware that the bereaved person is not operating on all cylinders and is going to forget things. That doesn't mean they are mentally unstable or have long-term brain damage; they just need to heal and must be given the time and support to do so. But at the time, lacking that knowledge, I was simply terrified.

For Joe, who was running a worldwide operation, who was required to be "on" 24-7, and who had people all over the globe depending on his decisions, there were many times when he simply wasn't able to work at full capacity. He had quite a few episodes where he would be sitting at his desk, reading something or working on something, and he would find that he couldn't retain any information. His mind was just somewhere else. Yet it was so busy trying to process David's loss that he was exhausted, as if he really was working grueling hours.

Gradually, I found that the best way to heal was to share

my experience. Doing so validated my feelings. Most people appreciated my sharing my story and were very supportive, and knowing that there *were* other people I wanted to be with helped me to find meaningful activities and groups that welcomed me. Not to mention that Joe and I still had a young daughter to raise—a blessing that kept us afloat.

As I became more receptive to the rest of the outside world, I began to recognize the things that could help restore me. As Elisabeth Kübler-Ross so eloquently observed, I would not be the same me, but I could be whole again.

This book stresses that palliative care is not only for the dying, and that is true. But serious and life-threatening illnesses can end in death, and when that happens, it's important to know there are resources to help you make your way back into the world. I hope you will use this chapter as a guide to discovering them. For example, unresolved feelings, guilt, confusion, and disturbing memories are all part of the grieving process, and a talented professional counselor can help you get through them. You'll discover the benefits of seeking help from such a person, and how to find one.

Being prepared for grief triggers, like anniversaries, birthday, and holidays, is another facet of life after goodbye. You can use these events as opportunities for special new traditions that honor the memory of your loved one; this chapter offers diverse ideas to consider. I found tremendous comfort in meeting with other parents who had lost a teenager, and in discussing ways to help newly diagnosed teens and their parents. This work led me, eventually, to discover palliative care, the part of health care that is now my passion and one of the ways I honor my son's memory.

Throughout this book, we've explored how palliative care for patients is fundamentally about improving their quality of life. In a similar sense, palliative care for survivors is about trying to improve their quality of life even as they're struggling with grief. If palliative care for the patient helps them to feel as if they have some control over their destiny, the same principles apply to the grieving process, even if the ill person ends up losing the battle. Others' lives continue, and a road map for getting through the pain and rebuilding can be invaluable.

Grief might feel embarrassing, but it doesn't have to be. I encourage you to accept it and simply excuse yourself. If you want to share what you are going through, you're welcome to, but you don't have to explain yourself if you don't want to. While none of us welcomes grief into our lives, it is an experience from which we can learn and grow, gaining new insights into our spirituality, and growing in our compassion. See it as a journey. I like to remind myself of what Winston Churchill once said: "The only way out is through."

THE SIX STAGES OF GRIEF

You may be familiar with the Kübler-Ross model, which proposes that humans go through five stages of grief: denial, anger, bargaining, depression, and acceptance. Although Kübler-Ross originally claimed that these stages occur in that particular sequence, she later recanted, noting that they can happen in any order. My personal experience has shown me that the latter definition is more accurate: You might start off with denial and then you go straight to depression, then back to bargaining. As grief expert Terri Daniel explains, grief is simply not a linear process: "You're sad, you're crying, you can't get out of bed. You're angry. That's loss. Then you get out of bed and you go write in your journal and take a walk in nature—that's restoration. Back and forth, back and forth. As long as you're moving between those two focuses all the time and you're not stagnant, you're gonna be fine."[2]

The book that Kübler-Ross cowrote with grief counselor David Kessler, *Finding Meaning: The Sixth Stage of Grief*, introduces the idea that "each person's grief is as unique as their fingerprint. But what everyone has in common is that no matter how they grieve, they share a need for their grief to be witnessed. That doesn't mean needing someone to try to lessen it or reframe it for them. The need is for someone to be fully present to the magnitude of their loss without trying to point out the silver lining." The book was inspired by the sudden death of Kessler's twenty-one-year-old son, after which, Kessler said, "I knew I couldn't and wouldn't stop at acceptance. There had to be something more." For him, "more" meant "meaning," which he calls the sixth stage of grief, "where the healing often resides," and which can help to ease our suffering.[3] Viktor Frankl would agree—his argument that people can find meaning in even the bleakest situations dovetails perfectly with Kessler's thinking.

TIPS FOR COPING

During the last six months of David's life, I was on a constant roller-coaster ride of life-and-death scenarios. I found that the only way I could get through it was to compartmentalize my life in a way that allowed me to block out everything that was going on in any environment besides the one I was in at any given moment. But after David died, all the pain I had been putting off and ignoring came rushing back in, and then I had to focus on healing, both physically and mentally. For me, that included not only a grief counselor but also for a period of time seeing a psychologist. As I mentioned at the beginning of this chapter, my grief for the first few years after David died controlled me, not the other way around. Now, I understand how many tools are at our disposal to help us feel as if we're managing our grief, rather than just letting it consume us.

When we moved to London after David died, my whole purpose in relocating was to be able to grieve on my own terms and at my own pace. When we lived in Connecticut, every activity and interaction after David's death felt forced. Everyone constantly reminded me of our loss. It was too painful. But in London I learned about the Teenage Cancer Trust, a UK charity that provides support and specialized nursing care for young people with cancer. When I got involved with that organization, I was surrounded by professionals or parents who had also lost teenagers. Meeting these other bereaved parents, who could empathize with what I was going through, felt deeply comforting, and the fact that we were all working together toward common goals was inspiring and energizing. In his books, Viktor Frankl talks about how the only way to grow is through pain. When I got really interested in Frankl, Joe said, "Be an advocate. What did you learn? How can you help others do something meaningful through sharing your experience?" Through the Teenage Cancer Trust, I discovered that sometimes an altruistic gesture is a wonderful way to make yourself feel better at the same time you're benefiting others.

Soon after that, I also joined an expat women's club. We'd go on trips together, and people would inevitably ask me, "What brought you to London?" How much I chose to share depended on the person who asked the question. If they seemed like someone I could feel comfortable opening up to, I'd say, "We moved here because we lost a child and we just needed a new beginning." Depending on how they responded, I would share more. I found my friendships with these women very healing. They were so supportive. But it was a process. Joe didn't feel the same way, nor did Sarah. I've always been the most social person in our family; they didn't think their grief was anyone else's business. Besides, Joe was working so much in those days that most of his interpersonal dynamics with people centered on his job, not his personal life.

The point is, everybody has a different way of grieving and expressing grief, and everybody has a different personality in general. That means there is no one right way or wrong way to grieve. It's entirely subjective. Even within a couple or a family, all members might have radically different responses to a loved one's illness or death, and that's okay. You can't force yourself to be a certain way. You have to allow yourself the space to do whatever feels right to you in a particular scenario, and you also have to be respectful of the fact that other people in your family or your household may be completely different from you, even if it's hard to do so. "Families who had communication problems before the death and families who adhere to rigid roles for each member are apt to create or exacerbate problems in grieving," say Carolyn Jaffe and Carol Ehrlich, authors of *All Kinds of Love: Experiencing Hospice*. "Their patterns do not help the individual members, who need particularly to be able to communicate openly, and who must function despite the death-created loss of family role-structure. Flexibility of roles . . . would enhance everyone's adaptation."

The authors continue by advising families to "share an acknowledgement of the death and loss (which can perhaps occur when the group takes time to look through old photos and records), reorganize the family system, and reinvest in new relationships and life pursuits."[4]

Some bereaved people seem not to grieve at all. They just bottle up all their feelings and never communicate about them. When Sarah was in graduate school, one of her assignments was to go to some kind of support group. Sarah, because she had lost someone, went to a bereavement group whose participants had recently experienced the death of a loved one. The group had to go around the circle and explain whom they had lost. Even though Sarah was talking about an event that had happened eleven years earlier, she started to cry in the middle of telling her story. It took her by surprise. I said to her, "It's because you choose not to talk about it."

No matter what particular characteristics your grief takes on, if you live in denial of it, you may find yourself facing clinical depression and all kinds of other health issues. For people who don't deal with it, it usually comes back to haunt them somehow. You don't have to talk about it with everybody, but you have to process it—you have to give yourself space and time to heal, mentally and physically—so that it doesn't become toxic and backfire on you. Grief needs expression, so let it out somehow.

For me, a number of different tactics helped me to process David's loss. I read books on grief, resilience, and how to recover after a trauma. I listened to classical music all the time, because it soothed me. I also sought the help of a professional grief counselor and saw her twice a week for two years. Talking with her helped immeasurably. However, what works for one person may not work for another. Any number of healing practices might resonate with you if you are mourning the loss of a loved one. The point is to experiment until you find what works for you, and then use it to your advantage. Here are a few suggestions:

- Join a support group

- Start a meditation practice

- Paint, sculpt, draw, or make ceramics

- Take long walks in nature

- Journal

- Write a letter, poem, or song to your loved one

- Create a photo album of pictures that remind you of happy times together

- Come up with rituals to perform on specific days to commemorate events in the lost love one's life

Grieving can be exhausting. Following suggestions like the ones below, from the Cleveland Clinic, will enable you to get the opportunities for rest and recuperation that you will desperately need if you are mourning the loss of a loved one:

- **Accept some loneliness:** If you feel lonely during the grieving process, know that it's normal, but also avoid becoming too comfortable in your loneliness. Find sources of support who will accept that everyone grieves differently and on different timelines.

- **Choose good company:** Seek out friends, old or new, who have been aggrieved themselves and who can provide companionship without burdening you by asking you for more than you can give. I shared my experience only with people I had a true bond with. As I started emerging from my shell, I slowly started sharing my experience with others, if they were willing to hear it.

- **Be gentle with yourself:** Avoid criticizing yourself for being a grieving person; realize that your grief is part of who you are right now (but may not be forever).

- **Embrace all emotions:** Realize that your feelings will happen whether you want them to or not. All you can do is let them pass, "like waves in the ocean or clouds in the sky."

- **Get extra rest:** "Physical and emotional exhaustion is common. You will need more rest than usual." After David died, I had to take a nap every afternoon, and not a short one—I would sleep for an hour and a half. That was just what my mind required at the time to process its emotional and physical overload.

- **Set a regular sleep schedule:** Go to bed and wake up at the same time every day. Rest when you need to, but avoid oversleeping.

- **Move your body:** Make a point of being active for part of every day, even if you don't feel like it and even if it's only for a few minutes. Try spending as much of your active time as possible outdoors.

- **Talk to your doctor:** Share with your primary care doctor that you are grieving, so that they can facilitate your physical and mental well-being.

- **Keep structure in your day:** Avoid falling into a rut by continuing to engage in the basic day-to-day activities you used to do to. Even if you don't feel motivated to get out of bed, change out of your pajamas, brush your teeth, or eat a meal, force yourself to do so.

- **Set goals:** "Set small, reachable, short-term goals so that you don't get overwhelmed."

- **Make a list of daily activities:** Getting into this habit can help you to keep track of what you need to do, especially if your grief is distracting you from being as organized as you usually are.

- **Be cautious:** Avoid making any significant life decisions while you are actively grieving.

- **Take care of your inner needs:** "Find time, whether through a spiritual practice or a creative outlet, to connect to things that give you inspiration and help you maintain your sense of meaning and purpose."[5]

Most of all, be patient with yourself as you take the time you need to heal. Give yourself permission to do what your body and mind are telling you to do. There's no rule that says you have to jump back into life as you knew it—you're never going to be the same person again. But eventually, you can still be someone who experiences moments of peace and even joy.

PAYING TRIBUTE

One of the most healing concepts that I discovered, thanks to a friend who visited us while we lived in London, was paying tribute to a lost loved one. My family's first tribute to David was a toy closet on the pediatric unit of a hospital that I worked at for many years. That gesture set in motion other, more significant future philanthropic endeavors for our family, including the Kanarek Family Foundation. Honoring his memory through the projects we do always makes me feel closer to David. Every time I do a project and wonder if I'm doing the right thing, I usually get goose bumps, and I take that as validation that David wants me to go on. It's as if he's giving me his stamp of approval.

Whether you erect a bench in memory of someone in a beautiful place, make a donation to a charitable cause that the person was passionate about, or do something entirely unique, it's a way to ultimately celebrate the life of the lost loved one in whatever way feels right to you and whatever way honors that person's memory best.

Virtually every day, something I say or do triggers a memory of David. His body may not be with us, but my family is keeping his spirit and his personality alive by continually talking about him and keeping our memories of him fresh—or imagining how he would react in certain situations. For example, maybe we drive to a beautiful place where David didn't get to go while he was alive, and we all look at each other and say, "David would love it here." It's a way of bringing him into the situation that's positive and healing for all of us.

Memories don't all have to be happy to ease your pain. Some of them can be idiosyncratic or even sad. For example, David thought the store Hammacher Schlemmer had a funny name, and it always made him laugh out loud. Joe and I bought several items from the company. To this day, every time a new catalog arrives, we look through it and smile. It's not funny for anybody else, but it's funny for us. It reminds us of David's unique quirks and gives us an opportunity to laugh with him again.

FINAL THOUGHTS

Paul J. Moon, PhD, author of numerous books and articles on grief and dying, says,

> Grief and palliative care are interrelated and perhaps mutually inclusive. Conceptually and practically, grief intimately relates to palliative care, as both domains regard the phenomena of loss, suffering, and a desire for abatement of pain burden. Moreover, the notions of palliative care and grief may be construed as being mutually inclusive in terms of one cueing the other. Indeed it is not easy to imagine a palliative care scenario where no trace of tacit or explicit grief is evidenced. In the same, it is deemed difficult to postulate a grief-striking condition where some degree of palliation would not be sought.[6]

Throughout this book, I have sought to underscore the many branches of palliative care and the ways in which they are interrelated. The subject of grief is no different. This chapter includes tips that I intend to be broadly helpful for people who are grieving and who are striving to recover improved quality of life. If you have lost a loved one, you will never be the same, and your pain won't ever disappear, but you *can* have a support network and coping tools at your disposal. I want people who are going through what I've experienced to finish this book and think, *I feel better knowing that countless others have been through this and that I now have some tools for rebuilding my life in a way that honors the person I lost but also makes me more fulfilled and able to move through each day with less pain and more ease.*

Many of the suggestions in this chapter fall into the category of self-directed kindness and gentleness. You should also be good to your living friends and family and be present in and cognizant of both the special and the everyday moments you have together. Eventually, you will realize that while the pain of someone's death never goes away entirely, you can learn how to manage it. As the aforementioned grief expert Terri Daniel tells it, "I like to say, 'Hello, grief. . . . I don't want you to be here, but I'm going to make friends with you because I can't get rid of you. So come on in and sit with me, and I will be your friend.' That's how you heal. That's how it strengthens you."[7]

Over time, I have learned to focus on all my memories of David and all the special time our family spent together. I have learned to accept what happened but also to work on making things better for today and tomorrow. Most of our loved ones who have died wouldn't want us to be pained for too long. They'd want us to move forward, especially when finding peace doesn't mean we have to forget the person we lost, as the poem below so beautifully illuminates.

Immortality
Clare Harner, 1909–1977

Do not stand
By my grave, and weep.
I am not there,
I do not sleep—
I am the thousand winds that blow
I am the diamond glints in snow
I am the sunlight on ripened grain,
I am the gentle, autumn rain.
As you awake with morning's hush,
I am the swift, up-flinging rush
Of quiet birds in circling flight,

I am the day transcending night.
Do not stand
By my grave, and cry—
I am not there,
I did not die.

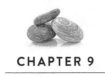

CHAPTER 9

Making Palliative Care Mainstream

WHAT LEGISLATORS, PHILANTHROPISTS, EDUCATORS, AND YOU CAN DO

*I often say now I don't have any choice whether or not
I have Parkinson's, but surrounding that non-choice
are a million other choices that I can make.*

—MICHAEL J. FOX, ACTOR, AUTHOR, FILM PRODUCER,
AND ACTIVIST FOR PARKINSON'S DISEASE

We know now that palliative care has been a recognized medical specialty in the United States since 2006 and that it is effective at helping people with a serious or life-threatening illness live longer, enjoy an optimal quality of life, avoid emergency room visits and hospitalization, and spend less money on care. Why, then, is it not a readily available offering in mainstream modern American medicine? What would it take to make that happen?

Making palliative care mainstream requires a multifaceted approach. We need to

1. convince legislators at the state and federal levels of the need to pass laws that make palliative care more accessible;

2. support philanthropic and other stakeholders seeking to invest in the advancement of palliative care;

3. ensure that nursing schools include palliative care in their curricula and clinical experiences, and make palliative care nursing a specialty;

4. cultivate leaders in the palliative care field;

5. introduce all health care students to the role of palliative care early in their education and promote and cultivate this area of specialization; and

6. establish priorities for the future.

Until palliative care is fully utilized within the US health care system, legislation, philanthropy, and activism are needed to propel it forward. This may seem like a tall order, but it can be done. In this chapter, I'll unpack the many branches of society that are currently working toward making palliative care more visible, more accessible, and less expensive for patients and health care providers alike.

LEGISLATION

In 1996, after concerted efforts by physicians, legislators, patients and their family members, and various psychiatric organizations, the Mental Health Parity Act (MHPA) was enacted. MHPA requires health insurance plans to offer the same annual or lifetime payment coverage on care for mental health as they do for medical and surgical care. Prior to MHPA, insurers were *not* required to cover mental health care; access to treatment was, therefore, limited at best, and more patients ended up seeking care in emergency rooms—a costly and ineffective scenario.

The Mental Health Parity Act came into being thanks to letter-writing campaigns, testimony by physicians and patients before the US Senate, and patients and families sharing their stories with news outlets. This success story on the mental health front should inspire those of us who want palliative care to gain similar governmental recognition in the United States. We *can* achieve it, but we have to start educating ourselves today about what the legal landscape looks like, and we have to align ourselves with the right groups and causes.

One highly worthwhile initiative to support is the Comprehensive Care Caucus, launched in 2019 by a group of US senators dedicated to passing legislation like the Provider Training in Palliative Care Act, which seeks to officially recognize palliative care as an eligible primary care service; the Rural Access to Hospice Act, which allows federally qualified health centers and rural health centers to receive payment for hospice services while acting as attending physicians for elderly rural patients who trust them; and the Palliative Care and Hospice Education and Training Act (PCHETA), which will "establish fellowship programs within new palliative care and hospice education centers to provide short-term, intensive training on palliative care and hospice . . . for medical school faculty, as well as other educators in health care fields such as nursing, pharmacy, social work, and chaplaincy."[1] Another excellent advocacy group is the Washington, DC–based Hospice Action Network, which is "dedicated to preserving and expanding access to hospice and palliative care in America, particularly by establishing an ongoing and widespread presence on Capitol Hill and "mobilizing a growing network of . . . advocates throughout the nation."[2]

Many individual states are also getting actively involved in the cause, proposing legislation and executive orders designed to assess their palliative care practices. Florida TaxWatch, for example, is pushing for the Florida legislature to develop a regulatory framework for palliative care, one that both protects patients and avoids overregulation. In 2019, New Jersey governor Phil Murphy passed a bill establishing a state advisory council on palliative care that will make information on palliative care more available to the public. Massachusetts passed Bill S 2400 in 2012, requiring hospitals, skilled-nursing and assisted-living facilities, and other medical centers to identify patients whom palliative care could benefit and to inform them of its availability. The Massachusetts Department of Public Health also sponsors the Pediatric Palliative Care Network, which provides palliative care services and quality-of-life improvements to children under age eighteen who have a terminal diagnosis, as well as their families. And in 2017, Virginia senator Mark Warner sponsored the Patient Choice and QualityCare Act, which proposes to increase patients' awareness of and access to advance care planning.

As of 2019, US states are fortunate to have a State Leadership Council on Palliative Care, convened jointly by the National Academy for State Health Policy and the John A. Hartford Foundation, examining the challenges they face in integrating palliative care across the health care field and educating both patients and providers about its benefits. The council has made recommendations, based on its findings, that include educating the public, health care providers, and policy makers about the value of palliative care and removing stigmas surrounding the concept; establishing strict state-by-state definitions of palliative care that help to distinguish it from hospice care; identifying best practices; building workforce capacity; and making palliative care available to Medicaid beneficiaries nationwide.[3]

These are only a handful of the plethora of legal efforts currently underway in the pro–palliative care arena. Their proliferation is heartening, but we cannot become complacent. Remember, a bill proposed is not the same as a bill passed, and even of the legislation that has been approved, not all has an enforcement mechanism or funding for implementation and evaluation. That is why we must continue to unite our voices and use our words to advocate for the benefits of palliative care across the nation, among lawmakers, attorneys, hospitals, health insurance companies, and society at large.

PHILANTHROPY

Philanthropy is the current backbone of palliative care activities. It can catalyze increased training and funding, as well as more continuing medical education, in the palliative care realm. It can also draw attention to palliative care as a discipline and educate the public about the field's current challenges and opportunities for improvement.

Although we need to recruit more philanthropists who are committed to supporting the growth of palliative care in the United States, numerous organizations are doing good work on this front already, including the Cambia Health Foundation and its Palliative Care Center of Excellence. The center is focused on "giving every patient with serious illness access to high-quality palliative care focused on relieving symptoms, maximizing quality of life, and ensuring care that concentrates on patients' goals," and to seeing "that palliative care has an integral and prominent role in health care—regionally, nationally and internationally—for seriously ill patients and their families." Cambia is a strong source of institutional support as well, teaching hospitals and other facilities building palliative care programs how to do so most effectively, as well as educating physicians, nurses, social workers, chaplains, and others on how best to deliver palliative care to patients. This last point of interest aims to rectify the low provider-to-patient ratio of about one palliative care medical professional for every 1,200 people with a serious illness.[4] Since 2009, the Cambia Health Foundation has invested more than $30 million in palliative care awareness, access, and quality and, in 2014, started the Sojourns Scholar Leadership Program to develop leaders in the field of palliative care nationwide.[5]

The Robert Wood Johnson Foundation, the largest public-health philanthropy in the United States, is another standout in this area. Dedicated to "building a Culture of Health that provides everyone in America a fair and just opportunity for health and well-being," the foundation developed a national program called Promoting Excellence in End-of Life Care.[6] In 2006, that program funded twenty-two demonstration projects in a wide variety of settings to test out innovative models of palliative care that could address deficiencies in the existing palliative care system, and determined that "it is possible to expand access to palliative services and improve quality of care in ways that are financially feasible and acceptable to patients, families, clinicians, administrators, and payers."[7]

The John A. Hartford Foundation (JAHF), mentioned earlier in this chapter, is a long-standing grant funder of the Center to Advance Palliative Care (CAPC) and also offers grant-based support for a handful of important initiatives, including National POLST (physician orders for life-sustaining treatment), an effort to standardize the POLST process nationwide, and the palliative care–based public-engagement initiative the Conversation Project.

As the elderly population in the United States grows, so does the need for palliative care, and so, too, will the need for funding sources. Philanthropic foundations like these are a crucial part of the equation, as they can supplement federal and state governments' and the health care sector's fiscal support of palliative care clinical services, research, and education.

NURSING EDUCATION

We talked in chapter 2 about the importance of expanding medical school curricula to include emphasis on palliative care, but nursing schools may be an even more significant forum for such changes. Nurses are the largest sector of health care professionals (exceeding four million in the United States, as of 2020), and those who spend the most time caring for seriously ill patients and their loved ones.[8] As the number of elderly and ill people in the United States continues to rise, and as terminal illnesses become more complex, nurses will be called upon more and more frequently to use core palliative care skills to interact with their patients and with the other members of medical teams. Thus, as Betty Ferrell, RN, and her colleagues note, "Future nurses must be able to help patients manage serious illness and its associated symptoms across the disease trajectory; communicate effectively and compassionately with patients, families, and the health care team; and provide psychosocial and spiritual support during care transitions and the bereavement period."[9] And in order for all this to happen, palliative care training simply must be part of every nursing school's curriculum.

In 2016, the American Nurses Association and the Hospice & Palliative Nurses Association collaborated to develop a Call for Action: Nurses Lead and Transform Palliative Care. Their recommendations include adopting End-of-Life Nursing Education Consortium (ELNEC) curricula as a standard for primary palliative care education for prelicensure, graduate, doctoral, continuing education, practical nurses, and advance practice nurses. Rose Virani and Betty Ferrell cofounded ELNEC, which is dedicated to educating nurses about palliative care and end-of-life patients' needs. This program is a gold mine of information for educators, and nursing schools are catching on. Since the first ELNEC training, in 2001, more than one hundred countries have requested the curriculum, which

> begins with an overview of why improving palliative and end-of-life care through a holistic and interdisciplinary approach is a necessary part of quality nursing. Subsequent modules cover the assessment and management of pain, particularly at the end of life; management of symptoms, including those experienced during advanced disease; ethical and legal issues; cultural and spiritual assessment

and care; effective communication with patients, family members, and the interdisciplinary team—a key focus of the program; loss and grief for patients, families, nurses, and other caregivers; and preparing for and administering care at the time of death. . . . [The program also] includes training on handling divisions between what family members may want for the patient and what patients want for themselves.[10]

In 2015, ELNEC received a grant from the Cambia Health Foundation to review, among other endeavors, the current state of palliative care undergraduate nursing education and current undergraduate nursing textbooks. As of 2016, more than one hundred textbooks focusing on hospice and palliative care existed, and new ones continue to be released, yet no regulatory organization is requiring faculty and students at nursing schools to read this literature. This oversight has a direct impact not only on nursing education but also, and perhaps more important, on patients themselves, who are ending up with nurses who do not always have the tools they need to navigate difficult discussions, facilitate interdisciplinary communication, or simply even be present in whatever way patients need them to be.

On a more productive note, another outcome of ELNEC's Cambia grant was a summit held in 2015 at which select faculty members from US nursing schools and leaders in the palliative nursing movement met to update a 1998 report called *Peaceful Death*, by the American Association of Colleges of Nursing (AACN), which listed the competencies all nurses were expected to have in order to provide effective end-of-life care. The summit participants' revisions resulted in *Palliative Competencies and Recommendations for Educating Undergraduate Nursing Students* (CARES), which recognizes the centrality of palliative care in nursing education and which is now the gold standard for that realm.[11]

So many interrelated circumstances make the need for palliative care nursing education more critical now than it has ever been before. Even nurses themselves are vocal about their desire for more training. In one extensive study of Midwestern registered nurses, participants described their wish to empower patients and families in end-of-life scenarios, as well as their challenges in areas such as offering palliative care in a timely manner, being a go-between for patients and health care providers or for patients and their families, and advocating for patients who needed adjustments in their pain medication. Ultimately, the study concluded that the nurses who participated did not meet the National Consensus Project's (NCP's) criteria for quality palliative care. Areas for improvement included "palliative assessments and care planning, symptom management beyond pain, psychological assessments and recognizing when mental health specialists are needed, family-focused care in times of conflict, and recognizing when a patient would benefit from hospice earlier in the illness trajectory."[12] Imagine how different NCP's impression might have been had these nurses had early access to up-to-date textbooks, to CARES, and to teachers dedicated to shepherding them through the complicated palliative care landscape. Imagine how much more caring and coordinated the entire health care industry could be if we populated it with graduates of medical and nursing schools who knew exactly how to comfort, to guide, and to add value in end-of-life scenarios before they even started their first jobs in their field. This is the crux of our national need for palliative care education. This is where tomorrow's nurses need to be guided.

LEADERSHIP

Cambia Health Foundation President Peggy Maguire and distinguished palliative care physician Steven Pantilat, of UCSF

Medical Center in San Francisco, have a heartfelt call to action regarding the need for palliative care leaders:

> The future of [palliative care] . . . rests on our ability to build a strong palliative care workforce. . . . It is essential to identify, develop, and promote leaders . . . who will serve as mentors in the development of other clinicians and who will become the future educators, researchers, and policy champions in the field. Weaving the discipline into the fabric of our evolving health care system and into the community will require leaders who can develop person- and family-oriented solutions, advance public policy, train generalist and specialist clinicians, and drive sustainable system change.[13]

The truth is, nurses are the real pioneers in this space. A doctor's job is to deal with patients' diseases; a nurse's job is to deal with the patients' well-being. You can dress up their roles in a thousand different ways, but that is the essence of why I envision palliative care as largely the domain of nurses.

When I got involved with the Teenage Cancer Trust (TCT), a registered charity in London that builds inpatient cancer units for teenagers, it was the first organization I participated in while I was still grieving David's loss. I expressed to the staff there that I really wanted to help those parents who had just found out their teens were diagnosed. While I was there, I met a nurse counselor, Vikky Riley, who dealt strictly with palliative care for teenagers who were dying. She and I quickly became friends, and when the TCT realized how well we worked together, it hosted an international conference on adolescent oncology where I spoke as the parent and she spoke as the nurse to health care professionals to highlight the need for more professionals like her in the health care system.

Ultimately, that presentation was published as a chapter in a book called *Cancer and the Adolescent*.[14] I gave an autographed copy to the chair of pediatrics at Memorial Sloan Kettering Cancer Center, where David received cancer treatment. I said, "I want you to know that it's going to be nurses who are going to be making palliative care a top priority and leading the field."

He looked at me and he chuckled. He said, "Oh, no, no, no."

I said, "Do you want to make a bet?" Well, I never got to find out whether I won, as the doctor has since retired, but when I spoke to Diane Meier, director emerita of CAPC, about the same subject, she implied that I was on the right track. "We will never have enough physicians going into this specialty," she told me. It's not a money maker. It's emotionally taxing. It's a twenty-four-hour-a-day job. For all of these reasons, plus the fact that physicians are often ill equipped or not trained sufficiently to deliver bad news, it's the nurses, not the doctors, who are really stepping up when it comes to palliative care leadership—and leadership is everything.

What does the strongest form of palliative care leadership look like? It looks like Constance Dahlin, MSN, director of professional practice at the Hospice & Palliative Nurses Association, palliative nurse practitioner, and CAPC consultant, who has emerged as a front-runner in this space. According to Dahlin, good leadership must encompass four areas of focus. "Palliative leadership in education assures development in palliative knowledge, attitudes, and skills. Palliative care leadership in clinical practice promotes excellence and evidence-based practice in delivery of quality care. Palliative care leadership in research fosters the continued development and maturity of the evidence to support and grow the specialty. Palliative leadership in policy and advocacy furthers changes in health care, delivery, and access."[15] It also means doing the right thing, having a vision, using critical-thinking skills, handling conflict negotiation, and taking a healthy team approach that respects various perspectives. Dahlin makes a case for shared, distributed leadership in lieu of an individual leader (who can quickly turn into a dictator under the wrong circumstances), and for interdisciplinary teams that are accountable to and can speak for each other. The traits of teams with a strong leadership culture, she emphasizes, are universal engagement, a shared vision, equality, honesty, and consistency of care and process.[16]

Unfortunately, dedicated palliative care leadership training facilities are few and far between. As of 2019, the American Academy of Hospice and Palliative Medicine was the only professional palliative care organization to offer aspiring leaders such an option. Other noteworthy programs are cropping up, including the National Hospice and Palliative Care Organization, which hosts a leadership and management conference centering on administrators, and CAPC, whose national initiative Palliative Care Leadership Centers seek to innovate health care through palliative care program design, growth, and sustainability.[17] And a cause that is especially near to my own heart is the Kanarek Center for Palliative Care Nursing Education at Fairfield University in Connecticut, which my family established in 2017 to help ready nursing students for palliative care leadership by offering them a comprehensive curriculum in the field.

A general dearth of academic choices isn't the only obstacle that nurses, the most logical demographic to take up the leadership mantle, face. Another issue is internal politics within care teams. Although, as we have discussed, physicians are often not the most qualified people to lead a care team because of the limits of their own training, they sometimes hesitate to delegate positions of authority to nurses, even when they might thrive in a leadership role, and when successful palliative care leadership depends on all members' being able to transform patient care. By the same token, some nurses may be reluctant to accept a leadership position because their traditional training has taught them that someone else is usually going to be in charge.[18]

In addition, some care teams are simply not clear about where nurses fit into the palliative care equation and thus do not encourage nurses to act in a leadership capacity. Nurses also run the risk of feeling as though they exist "in between" doctors and patients and do not have full respect or trust from either camp.

My hope is that this book will help to rectify some of these misconceptions, highlight the need for more leadership training programs, and encourage nurses to emerge as the leaders they are meant to be within the palliative care discipline. Despite the hindrances they face, Jane Phillips, president of Palliative Care Nurses Australia, agrees that nurses are "ideally placed to address each individual person's palliative care needs and to innovate to ensure that the physical, psychological, emotional, spiritual, and informational aspects of a person with palliative care needs are appropriately addressed. As nurses, we can leverage our diverse roles, caring for people within our acute care hospitals, nursing homes, prisons, or homes for people with disabilities, to shape palliative care practice."[19]

We've already talked briefly about whole-person care. As the providers in hospital settings and other medical facilities who have the most frequent interpersonal exchanges with patients on any given day, nurses embody this kind of care. They have the foundation they need to become visionaries and guides in palliative care; now we just need to give them the resources, the confidence, and the voices to realize their potential.

PALLIATIVE CARE STAKEHOLDERS

As the palliative care field grows, so too does interest from a wide variety of stakeholders in the industry, including individuals (health care providers, policy makers, business leaders, even patients themselves) and institutions (hospitals, home care settings, palliative care centers, long-term care centers, and rehabilitation centers) that recognize the benefits of palliative care to patients, as well as the associated cost savings. Of the 2.6 million people who died in the United States in 2014, eight of ten were people on Medicare, and spending on Medicare beneficiaries in their last year of life accounts for about 25 percent of total Medicare spending on beneficiaries sixty-five and older, many of whom "often use costly services, including inpatient hospitalizations, post-acute care, and hospice, in the year leading up to their death."[20]

To mitigate this level of gross expenditure, private investors are seeking ways to increase value wherever they can find it. For example, Trinity Health, which provides palliative care across twenty-two US states, has implemented CAPC's evidence-based tools and best-practice guidelines across all of its ninety-two hospitals, using CAPC's online training curriculum to standardize palliative care capacity to ensure all-patient access and train clinicians and first-year residents in palliative care core competencies.[21] And OSF HealthCare, an integrated health care network serving patients of all ages across Illinois and Michigan, asked the inpatient operating unit at each of its facilities to develop a palliative care team in-house—a decision that has led not only to bottom-line savings but also to shorter hospital stays.[22]

Former CAPC director Diane Meier explains, "Hospitals are able to invest in hospital palliative care teams because they can't afford not to. . . . The more risk-bearing and movement towards value instead of volume a community or a region or a health system is doing, the higher the likelihood that they are investing resources and scaling access to palliative care."[23] Although she also argues that for-profit investors are not a long-term financial solution, and rather supports the idea of health care systems' building capacity and addressing the lack of palliative care–specific training in the medical workforce, even the companies—Trinity, OSF, VITAS Healthcare, and Senior Care Centers of America, among others—that are undoubtedly taking advantage of a big-money market are still helping to shine a spotlight on all the advantages of palliative care. In this respect, stakeholders are just as important as any other part of the equation.

PRIORITIES FOR THE FUTURE

So, what do we do with all this information? Where do we go from here?

First, knowledge is power. One of our top objectives for the future should be investing in more palliative care research. In 2015, a team of researchers identified the following topics as the most critical for exploration: needs of family caregivers; patients' perspectives; culture and ethnicity; patient-family or patient-provider decision making and communication; perspectives of professional caregivers; patients' emotional and psychological status; economic research and cost effectiveness; education, training, and curriculum development for health care providers; spirituality and existential issues; patterns of use, admittance, and referral; interdisciplinary approaches to delivering palliative care; and patients with conditions other than cancer.[24] The researchers underscored the importance of more rigorous research, as "there is widespread consensus that adequate scientific knowledge is lacking in many areas."[25]

Another critical area of focus is the integration of digitization and advanced technology, such as artificial intelligence (AI) and digital therapeutics (DTx), into palliative care and hospice care. The rapidly growing palliative care field is already understaffed and underresourced and will only become more so as patient need outpaces the number of specialists available. Researchers predict that digital technologies will provide an antidote by revolutionizing the way health care services are delivered. DTx are evidence-based health care products that use such technology as mobile apps, online platforms, and wearable devices to improve patient care. AI performs tasks that traditionally require human cognition.[26] Other services include telemedicine; automated speech, language, and image processing; and robotic caregivers.[27] Palliative care specialists are working diligently to identify how to harness the power of these groundbreaking tools in ways that make palliative care more effective, widespread, and innovative.

An attendant priority is, of course, how to preserve the humanity inherent in palliative care amid this digital revolution. Researchers Sheila Payne, Mark Tanner, and Sean Hughes note, "Among the mass of data generated, checkboxes and predefined answers that patients are invited to respond to, we can easily lose sense of the patient as an individual with their own life story, values, beliefs, and relationships. As the digital revolution in healthcare progresses, ensuring that the focus remains on the whole person, rather than their quantifiable parts, will probably be the greatest challenge of all." They also point out that data security, accuracy, and privacy will be paramount in circumstances in which doctors spend more time looking at patients' electronic health records than they do interacting with the patients themselves.[28] In an industry where so few practitioners make person-centered care the core of their business, we cannot allow the same fate to befall palliative care.

FINAL THOUGHTS

We in the United States are fortunate to have a robust and dedicated community of palliative care experts and cheerleaders who are working tirelessly to make advances in the field. However, the most important lesson I want you to glean from this chapter is that while palliative care awareness has come a long way, we must never stop continuing to enlighten people about it—and not just patients, hospitals, and insurance companies but legislators, attorneys, nonprofits and for-profits, private- and public-sector organizations. . . . The list feels nearly endless, but we cannot give up on reaching these audiences if we are to ensure that palliative care is available to all people who need it, *when* they need it—not just at the very end of their lives, but as soon as they receive a diagnosis. We can already envision a world where that happens; now we have to make it a reality.

EPILOGUE

David's Legacy

THE KANAREK FAMILY FOUNDATION

To live in hearts we leave behind is not to die.
—THOMAS CAMPBELL (1777–1844), POET

After my son's leukemia diagnosis in 1995, the medical treatments he underwent were the very best available at the time. However, David did not receive care that addressed his quality of life, his personal goals, his spirituality, or any of the other facets that made him the individual he was. Years later, when I learned about palliative care and all the ways in which it can help patients with a serious or life-threatening illness, as well as their family members and caregivers, I wished it had been offered to David and our family. His interaction with modern American medicine was disease-centered only, not—as is the hallmark of palliative care—patient- or person-centered care.

The more I discovered about the scope of palliative care, the more passionate I became about making coping with a serious illness a well-known part of mainstream medicine. As a mother who had lost her son, and as a health care professional myself, I could appreciate the value of an interdisciplinary team that addresses a patient's physical and psychological comforts, cultural traditions, social needs, spiritual questions, challenges with tasks of daily living, and more—and not just at the end of life or as a substitute for curative treatments, but for as long as they live with their illness. That was one of the unforgettable lessons I learned from my experience.

Seventeen years after David's death, I wrote an essay entitled "Life-Threatening Illness and a Mother's Emotional Journey: Lessons in Care" for the *Journal of Palliative Medicine*, in which I detailed my journey through losing David and the other meaningful insights that had emerged. Those reflections, which continued to resonate with me as I wrote this book, include the following:

- When David was hospitalized during and after his stem cell transplant, I learned how critical the psychological aspects of care are. Never underestimate the importance of addressing a patient's mental, emotional, and spiritual distress head-on—the earlier, the better.

- Continuity is a core goal of palliative care. Cultivate the team that is going to provide the most consistent, most well-rounded, most long-term support for you or your loved ones.

- Doctors, nurses, psychotherapists, social workers, chaplains, and other specialists should never stop learning, even after they have completed their formal training. Knowledge of the basics of advanced communication skills must be addressed in all areas of health care to provide the full scope of care—medical, physical, emotional, and spiritual—to patients and their families when they are most vulnerable.

- After my family relocated to London, four months after David's passing, I became involved with the Teenage Cancer Trust two years hence and knew I had found my voice. As I described in the introduction and chapter 9, not only was I able to share David's story with others, but I had an opportunity to give an extensive presentation, along with my nurse friend Vikky Riley, to health care providers about the unique needs of adolescents with cancer. If you are struggling with a loved one's diagnosis, identify whatever you need to do to reclaim your own voice, and use it for the greater good.[1]

Joe and I wanted to do something lasting and far-reaching to honor David's all-too-brief life, so, in 2006, we established the Kanarek Family Foundation. Its mission is to improve the quality of life of those affected by cancer or other life-threatening conditions through the promotion and integration of palliative care into all areas of American health care.

Since 2007, the foundation has helped support nursing education programs at Fairfield University by funding a Nursing Simulation Lab; underwriting a two-year initiative titled Nursing Curriculum Integration: Pediatric & Adolescent Palliative Care; and providing a significant grant to launch the award-winning Master of Science in Nursing Leadership program.

In 2011, the foundation funded a groundbreaking, five-year program at Memorial Sloan Kettering Cancer Center for the creation of an advanced communication skills module and simulation for nurse practitioners caring for pediatric patients and their families. As of 2021, a robust number of pediatric nurse practitioners have completed the program.

In 2017, the foundation opened the Kanarek Center for Palliative Care Nursing Education at Fairfield University Egan School of Nursing, an achievement that I initiated, launched, and continue to underwrite. In 2020, I began working with Christina Puchalski and Betty Ferrell, both of whom are featured in this book, to develop an interprofessional spiritual care education curriculum for pediatrics (ISPEC-PEDS). An ISPEC program for adults had already been established, but no one had highlighted the issues with pediatric patients yet.

All of these projects represent David's legacy. He may not have had the advantage of support that treats each patient as a whole person and that tends to the body, mind, and spirit. But as long as his story can enlighten other patients and their families, health care professionals, and the general public about palliative care, his soul will live on and continue to brighten countless lives, as it did when he was alive.

Serious illness may cut our lives short or alter them forever, but it doesn't have to define who we are or deprive us of the joy of living. If you or someone you love has received such a diagnosis, I hope this book has granted you moments of solace, of levity, of hope, of inspiration. But this is only the beginning of the fight. Palliative care continues to be little known and largely misunderstood, even within the medical community. We must continue to educate ourselves and each other about its many gifts so that all of us, when the time comes, can benefit. Each of us is a whole, complex person, and none of us deserves any less than care that recognizes the unique needs, questions, and desires that make us who we are.

Acknowledgments

The journey to the realization that I needed to write a book about palliative care was a long and arduous one. It began two years after my family and I relocated to London in 2000. I read in a local magazine about the Teenage Cancer Trust, a UK charity whose mission was to provide specialized care to young adults with cancer. The concept intrigued me, since nothing like this was available in the United States at the time. I met with the founders and staff and asked to become an active volunteer; I hoped that I could contribute suggestions on how to support parents of teens. Over several years, I met devoted health care professionals who wanted to improve the lives of teens battling this horrific disease. Through this charity, I realized I had a voice, as the mother of a child who had succumbed to cancer and as a nurse, to improve care. I am forever grateful that I had this opportunity to volunteer for this stellar organization. Thank you, Myrna, Adrian, and Simon!

After I returned to the United States, Dr. Eileen O'Shea, a professor of pediatric nursing at Fairfield University, my alma mater, introduced me to the concept of palliative care in 2008. I am eternally thankful for her guidance and friendship. She currently serves as the director of the Kanarek Center for Palliative Care in the Egan School of Nursing. After the center was opened and we began educating nurses and other health care professionals on what palliative care is, I soon realized that the public needed to learn about the multitude of its benefits for those with a serious illness. That was the number one reason I decided to write this book.

Amy Berman epitomizes what palliative care should and can be by sharing her own experience living with stage 4 breast cancer. She never ceases to amaze me with her elegance, insight, and wisdom.

Thank you to Dr. Betty Ferrell, PhD, RN; Diane Meier, MD; and Brynn Bowman for sharing their knowledge of, passion for, and steadfast support of palliative care. We have their tireless efforts to thank for continued progress in this field.

Christina Puchalski, MD, was a major influence in my realization of the concept of spiritual distress. For years, I struggled with trying to understand the changes in David's behavior when he was in strict isolation after his stem cell transplant. I had a sense that he was questioning his mortality, but when Christina described spiritual distress to a group of health care providers at a conference at Fairfield University, it was an aha moment for me. It finally addressed the many questions I had harbored for more than twenty years.

Rabbi M. J. Newman introduced me to the concept of spirituality in palliative care in a clinical setting. Her passion, commitment, and direction to patients never cease to amaze me. I am grateful to be her friend and mentee.

This book is a result of the guidance and unwavering support of Lisa Tener, Martha Murphy, and Annie Tucker, each a powerhouse of knowledge in the publishing field, and whose insight gave me the support I needed to produce this labor of love.

Thank you to Don Fehr, my literary agent, whom I have yet to meet face-to-face because of COVID. I am grateful for his support and his belief in this project.

A special thank-you is due to palliative care expert educator Sunita Puri for her tireless contributions to this field.

Lastly, and most importantly, to my family:

Sarah, you have grown to be a loving and wise woman. I know that the loss of your brother, David, changed your life immeasurably. You were five years old when he was diagnosed with leukemia and ten when he died. Soon after his death, we moved abroad, you started a new school midyear, and you had to make new friends in a new culture. It was a hard journey for you, but you came into your own and are thriving.

To the love of my life, Joe, my husband for more than forty years: This book is a part of you as much as it is of me. We collaborated through its entirety and had to rehash some difficult memories together. You have always been my biggest fan, no matter what project I undertook. Your love, unwavering support, guidance, and devotion are the greatest gifts I could hope for.

And to my dearest David: I hope that as you watch me "from above," you are proud of what I have accomplished in your memory. You would have been thirty-nine years old this year. Not a day goes by that I don't think of you and miss you. You were a courageous, witty, intelligent young man who was deeply loved. Your presence is always with me, and your father and I will continue to honor your memory. Please continue meeting me in my dreams.

Resources

American Academy of Hospice and Palliative Medicine: http://aahpmblog.org.

Commission on Law and Aging, American Bar Association, *Advance Directives: Counseling Guide for Lawyers*, 2018: www.americanbar.org/products/inv/brochure/346598312.

Education in Palliative and End-of-Life Care: www.bioethics.northwestern.edu/programs/epec.

End-of-Life Nursing Education Consortium (ELNEC): www.aacn.nche.edu/elnec.

Hospice & Palliative Nurses Association: https://advancingexpertcare.org.

National Academies of Sciences, Engineering, and Medicine
- *Health Literacy and Palliative Care: Workshop Summary*, 2016: http://nap.edu/21839.
- *Improving Palliative Care for Cancer*, 2001: http://nap.edu /catalog/10149/improving-palliative-care-for-cancer.
- *Integrating Health Care and Social Services for People with Serious Illnesses: Proceedings of a Workshop*, 2019: http:// nap.edu/25350.
- *Integrating the Patient and Caregiver Voice into Serious Illness Care: Proceedings of a Workshop*, 2017: http://nap.edu/24802.
- *Models and Strategies to Integrate Palliative Care Principles into Care for People with Serious Illness*, 2018: http://nap .edu/24908.

National Hospice and Palliative Care Organization: www.nhpco.org.

National Institute of Nursing Research: www.ninr.nih.gov /newsandinformation/conversationsmatter/conversations -matter-newportal#.VjzTIdKrS70.

Pallimed: www.pallimed.org.

Social Work Hospice and Palliative Care Network: www.swhpn.org.

VITALTalk: http://vitaltalk.org.

Resources for Patients

AARP and Caregiving Resource Center: www.aarp.org /caregiving.

Advance Health Care Directive Form: oag.ca.gov.

American Cancer Society: www.cancer.org/treatment/finding -and-paying-for-treatment/understanding-financial-and-legal -matters/advance-directives/types-of-advance-health-care -directives.html.

CaringBridge: www.caringbridge.org.

Caring Connections: www.nhpco.org/patients-and-caregivers.

CaringInfo: www.caringinfo.org.
CaringInfo, a program of the National Hospice and Palliative Care Organization, provides free resources to help people make decisions about services before a crisis.

Choosing Wisely: www.choosingwisely.org/patient-resources
/palliative-care.

The Conversation Project: https://theconversationproject.org.
Dedicated to helping people talk about their wishes for advance
care planning.

Courageous Parents Network: https://courageousparents
network.org.
Created by parents, for parents, to support, guide, and
strengthen families as they care for a seriously ill child, this
organization offers wisdom from fellow parents and pediatric
care providers to help people be the best parents they can be to
their children.

The Eldercare Locator: www.eldercare.gov.
This organization, a public service of the US Administration
on Aging, connects people to services for older adults and their
families.

Family Caregiver Alliance: https://caregiver.org/resource
/caregivers-count-too-toolkit.

Family Caregivers Providing Complex Chronic Care:
www.aarp.org/content/dam/aarp/research/public_policy
_institute/health/home-alone-family-caregivers-providing
-complex-chronic-care-rev-AARP-ppi-health.pdf.

Five Wishes: https://fivewishes.org/five-wishes.
Five Wishes is a comprehensive, person-centered advance-
care-planning program that offers health care providers a
proven, easy-to-use approach to having effective and compassionate conversations.

GeriPal: www.geripal.org.
GeriPal is a forum for discourse, recent news and research, and freethinking commentary. Its objectives are (1) to create an online community of interdisciplinary providers interested in geriatrics or palliative care; (2) to provide an open forum for the exchange of ideas and disruptive commentary that changes clinical practice and health care policy; and (3) to change the world.

Get Palliative Care: www.getpalliativecare.org.
Get Palliative Care is a website providing clear, comprehensive palliative care information for people living with a serious illness. The site is provided by the Center to Advance Palliative Care (CAPC).

Informed Patient Institute: www.informedpatientinstitute.org.
This organization rates websites to help people find doctors, hospitals, and/or nursing homes in their state, as well as tips about quality.

John Hartford Foundation: www.johnahartford.org.
The John Hartford Foundation is dedicated to improving the care of older adults and supports the spread of evidence-based models of care that can dramatically accelerate care improvements for them.

National Alliance for Caregiving: www.caregiving.org.

National Hospice and Palliative Care Organization: www.nhpco.org/palliative-care.

National Institute of Nursing Research

Pediatric:

www.ninr.nih.gov/newsandinformation/conversations
matter/conversationsmatter-patients.

General:

www.ninr.nih.gov/sites/files/docs/palliative-care
-brochure.pdf.

www.ninr.nih.gov/newsandinformation/what-is
-palliative-care.

www.ninr.nih.gov/researchandfunding/desp/oepcr.

National Palliative Care Research Center: www.npcrc.org.

National Resource on LGBT Aging: www.lgbtagingcenter.org.
This is the first and only technical assistance resource center
in the United States aimed at improving the quality of services
and supports offered to lesbian, gay, bisexual, and/or trans-
gender older adults.

Palliative Care Provider Directory: https://getpalliativecare
.org/provider-directory.
Get Palliative Care provides a full directory of all palliative
care providers by state and includes hospitals, nursing homes,
offices/clinics, and home care.

Palliative Care Research Cooperative Group:
https://palliativecareresearch.org.

Patient Rising: www.patientrising.org.
Patient Rising is dedicated to providing support and education
to those with chronic and life-threatening illnesses.

Tool Kit for Health Care Advance Planning, 3rd edition, 2020: www.americanbar.org/content/dam/aba/administrative /law_aging/2020-tool-kit-hcap.pdf.

US Department of Health & Human Services: www.nia.nih.gov /health/advance-care-planning-health-care-directives#what.

Popular Palliative Care Books

Mitch Albom, *Tuesdays with Morrie: An Old Man, A Young Man, and Life's Greatest Lesson*, New York: Doubleday, 1997.

Elizabeth Bailey, *The Patient's Checklist: 10 Simple Hospital Checklists to Keep You Safe, Sane, and Organized*, New York: Hachette, 2011.

Karen Whitley Bell, *Living at the End of Life: A Hospice Nurse Addresses the Most Common Questions*, New York: Sterling Ethos, 2010.

William S. Breitbart, *Individual Meaning-Centered Psychotherapy for Patients with Advanced Cancer: A Treatment Manual*, New York: Oxford University Press, 2014.

Katy Butler, *The Art of Dying Well: A Practical Guide to a Good End of Life*, New York: Scribner, 2019.

Ira Byock, *The Best Care Possible: A Physician's Quest to Transform Care through the End of Life*, New York: Avery Publishing, 2012.

Eric J. Cassell, *The Nature of Suffering and the Goals of Medicine*, New York: Oxford University Press, 1991.

Pema Chödrön, *When Things Fall Apart: Heart Advice for Difficult Times*, Boulder, CO: Shambhala Publications, 1997.

Susan R. Dolan and Audrey R. Vizzard, *The End-of-Life Advisor: Personal, Legal, and Medical Considerations for a Peaceful, Dignified Death*, New York: Kaplan Publishing, 2009.

David Dosa, *Making Rounds with Oscar: The Extraordinary Gift of an Ordinary Cat*, New York: Hyperion, 2009.

Norine Dresser and Fredda Wasserman, *Saying Goodbye to Someone You Love: Your Emotional Journey through End of Life and Grief*, New York: Demos Medical Publishing, 2010.

David B. Feldman and S. Andrew Lasher, Jr., *The End-of-Life Handbook: A Compassionate Guide to Connecting with and Caring for a Dying Loved One*, Oakland, CA: New Harbinger, 2007.

Sheri Fink, *Five Days at Memorial: Life and Death in a Storm-Ravaged Hospital*, New York: Crown Publishing, 2013.

Viktor Frankl, *Man's Search for Meaning*, Boston: Beacon Press, 1959.

Helen Garner, *The Spare Room*, New York: Henry Holt, 2008.

Atul Gawande, *Being Mortal: Medicine and What Matters in the End*, New York: Metropolitan Books, 2014.

Vivian E. Greenberg, *Children of a Certain Age: Adults and Their Aging Parents*, Lanham, MD: Lexington Books, 1994.

Christopher Hitchens, *Mortality*, New York: Hachette, 2012.

Paul Kalanithi, *When Breath Becomes Air*, New York: Random House, 2016.

Sharon R. Kaufman, *And a Time to Die: How American Hospitals Shape the End of Life*, New York: Scribner, 2005.

Christopher Kerr, *Death Is But a Dream: Finding Hope and Meaning at Life's End*, New York: Avery, 2020.

Elisabeth Kübler-Ross, *On Death and Dying*, New York: Scribner, 1969.

David Kuhl, *What Dying People Want: Practical Wisdom for the End of Life*, New York: PublicAffairs, 2002.

Harold S. Kushner, *When Bad Things Happen to Good People*, New York: Anchor Books, 1981.

Roi Livne, *Values at the End of Life: The Logic of Palliative Care*, Cambridge, MA: Harvard University Press, 2019.

Karen Macmillan, *A Caregiver's Guide: A Handbook about End-Of-Life Care*, Paris: Military and Hospitaller Order of St. Lazarus of Jerusalem, 2004.

Robert Martensen, *A Life Worth Living: A Doctor's Reflections on Illness in a High-Tech Era*, New York: Farrar, Straus and Giroux, 2008.

B. J. Miller and Shoshana Berger, *A Beginner's Guide to the End: Practical Advice for Living Life and Facing Death*, New York: Simon & Schuster, 2019.

Virginia Morris, *Talking about Death Won't Kill You*, New York: Workman, 2001.

Jo Myers, *Good to Go: A Guide to Preparing for the End of Life*, New York: Sterling, 2010.

Sherwin B. Nuland, *How We Die: Reflections on Life's Final Chapter*, New York: Vintage Books, 1995.

Tim O'Brien, *The Things They Carried*, New York: Houghton Mifflin, 1990.

Steven Pantilat, *Life after the Diagnosis: Expert Advice on Living Well with a Serious Illness for Patients and Caregivers*, Boston: Da Capo Press, 2017.

Nina Riggs, *The Bright Hour: A Memoir of Living and Dying*, New York: Simon & Schuster, 2017.

Elliott J. Rosen, *Families Facing Death: A Guide for Healthcare Professionals and Volunteers*, San Francisco: Jossey-Bass, 1998.

Cicely Saunders, Mary Baines, and Robert Dunlop, *Living with Dying: A Guide for Palliative Care*, New York: Oxford University Press, 1995.

Will Schwalbe, *The End of Your Life Book Club*, New York: Alfred A. Knopf, 2012.

Morrie Schwartz, *Morrie in His Own Words*, New York: Walker and Company, 1996.

Jessica Nutik Zitter, *Extreme Measures: Finding a Better Path to the End of Life*, New York: Avery, 2017.

Media

L'Chayim: Robin Kanarek (Transcending Loss): www.youtube
.com/watch?v=LDHFq5vfN10.
In May 2019, Rabbi Mark Golub, founder and host of the
Jewish Broadcasting Service (www.jbstv.org), hosted me in
a wide-ranging discussion about palliative care, my Jewish
background, my nursing background, and my experience
with David's illness.

GeriPal: geripal.org/p/geripal-podcast.html.
A podcast for healthcare professionals about geriatrics and
palliative care.

Graceful Passages: www.gracefulpassages.com/products
/graceful.html.
The two-CD gift book *Graceful Passages* offers compassion,
comfort, and emotional healing for people facing life-
threatening illness, grieving a loved one, or caring for our
soul. It includes messages shared by Elisabeth Kübler-Ross,
Ram Dass, Thich Nhat Hanh, Rabbi Zalman Schachter-
Shalomi, and other mentor guides.

National Public Radio: *Exploring Death in America*:
www.npr.org/programs/death.
This excellent, in-depth radio series provides resources, bibli-
ographies, transcripts, and audio recordings on a broad range
of end-of-life-related subjects.

New Dimensions: www.newdimensions.org.
New Dimensions Radio fosters the process of living a more
healthy life of mind, body, and spirit while deepening our connections to self, family, community, and the environment. Its

website features a selection of great shows on death and dying that have aired over the years.

On Our Own Terms: Moyers on Dying:
www.pbs.org/wnet/onourownterms.
This four-part video series from Bill Moyers crosses the country from hospitals to hospices to homes to capture some of the most intimate stories ever filmed and the most candid conversations ever shared with a television audience about end-of-life care. The Zen Hospice Project's volunteer program was featured in the first segment, "Living with Dying."

Sounds True: www.soundstrue.com.
Sounds True provides audio, video, and music for the inner life. This link will take you to a selection of the website's programs on death and dying.

With Eyes Open: www.pbs.org/witheyesopen.
KQED presented four half-hour companion shows to *On Our Own Terms*: honest discussions about caregiving, grief, difficult decisions, and what may lie beyond death. The first episode, "Mourning," was a conversation about loss, grief, and healing facilitated by the founder of the Zen Hospice Project and Metta Institute, Frank Ostaseski.

Notes

Introduction. David's Story
1. Atul Gawande, *Being Mortal: Medicine and What Matters in the End* (New York: Metropolitan Books, 2014), 187.
2. Gawande, *Being Mortal*, 259.

Chapter 1. What Is Palliative Care?
1. Timothy E. Quill and Amy P. Abernethy, "Generalist Plus Specialist Palliative Care—Creating a More Sustainable Model," *New England Journal of Medicine* 368, no. 13 (2013): 1173–75.
2. Quill and Abernethy, "Generalist Plus Specialist," 1173–75.
3. Betty Ferrell, "Ethical Perspectives on Pain and Suffering," *Pain Management Nursing* 6, no. 3 (2005): 83–90.
4. V. S. Periyakoil, H. C. Kraemer, and A. Noda, "Creation and the Empirical Validation of the Dignity Card-Sort Tool to Assess Factors Influencing Erosion of Dignity at Life's End," *Journal of Palliative Medicine* 12, no. 12 (2009): 1125–30.
5. Memorial Sloan Kettering Cancer Center, "Treating Cancer Pain," www.mskcc.org/cancer-care/diagnosis-treatment/symptom -management/palliative-care/pain-management/treating-pain.
6. Jae-A Lim et al., "Cognitive-Behavioral Therapy for Patients with Chronic Pain," *Medicine* 97, no. 23 (2018): e10867.
7. Mayo Clinic, "Pet Therapy: Animal as Healers," www.mayoclinic.org /healthy-lifestyle/consumer-health/in-depth/pet-therapy/art-20046342.
8. Priyanka Singh and Aditi Chaturvedi, "Complementary and Alternative Medicine in Cancer Pain Management: A Systematic Review," *Indian Journal of Palliative Care* 21, no. 1 (2015): 105–15.
9. Esmé Finlay, Michael W. Rabow, and Mary K. Buss, "Filling the Gap: Creating an Outpatient Palliative Care Program in Your Institution," *American Society of Clinical Oncology Educational Book* 38 (2018): 111–21.
10. Lisa Haney, "Palliative Care Specialists Can Reduce Your Pain and Speed Healing," *AARP Bulletin*, September 2018, www.aarp.org/health /conditions-treatments/info-2018/palliative-care-hospital-health-team .html.
11. National Hospice and Palliative Care Organization, "Palliative Care Overview," www.nhpco.org/palliativecare.
12. Cate Swannell, "Making Palliative Care about Quality of Life," *InSight+*, November 2021, https://insightplus.mja.com.au/2021/41/making -palliative-care-about-quality-of-life.
13. Jennifer S. Temel et al., "Effects of Early Integrative Palliative Care in Patients with Lung and GI Cancer: A Randomized Clinical Trial," *Journal of Clinical Oncology* 35, no. 8 (2017): 834–41.

14. Temel, "Effects of Early Integrative Palliative Care."
15. Haney, "Palliative Care Specialists."
16. Ariadne Labs, "Read Dr. Atul Gawande's Testimony before US Senate Special Committee on Aging on Serious Illness," www.ariadnelabs .org/2016/06/23/read-dr-atul-gawandes-testimony-before-u-s-senate -special-committee-aging-on-serious-illness/.
17. Atul Gawande, *Being Mortal: Medicine and What Matters in the End* (New York: Metropolitan Books, 2014), 147.

Chapter 2. Barriers to Palliative Care
1. Sunita Puri, *That Good Night: Life and Medicine in the Eleventh Hour* (New York: Viking, 2019), 10.
2. Center to Advance Palliative Care, "Serious Illness Strategies for Health Plans and Accountable Care Organizations," https://media.capc.org /filer_public/2c/69/2c69a0f0-c90f-43ac-893e-e90cd0438482/serious _illness_strategies_web.pdf.
3. Trevor Lane, Deepa Ramadurai, and Joseph Simonetti, "Public Awareness and Perceptions of Palliative and Comfort Care," *American Journal of Medicine* 132, no. 2 (2019): 129–31.
4. Lane, Ramadurai, and Simonetti, "Public Awareness and Perceptions."
5. Debra Bradley Ruder, "From Specialty to Shortage," *Harvard Magazine*, March–April 2015.
6. Lane, Ramadurai, and Simonetti, "Public Awareness and Perceptions"; Mark T. Hughes and Thomas J. Smith, "The Growth of Palliative Care in the United States," *Annual Review of Public Health* 35, no. 3 (2014): 459–75.
7. Hughes and Smith, "Growth of Palliative Care."
8. Jennifer Abbasi, "New Guidelines Aim to Expand Palliative Care Beyond Specialists," *Journal of the American Medical Association* 322, no. 3 (2019): 193–95.
9. Debra Bradley Ruder, "An Extra Layer of Care," *Harvard Magazine*, March–April 2015.
10. Center to Advance Palliative Care, "America's Care of Serious Illness," 2019, https://reportcard.capc.org.
11. Abbasi, "New Guidelines."
12. Kayla Sheehan, "Nourish the Roots: The Importance of Palliative Care Education in Medical School," Center to Advance Palliative Care, www .capc.org/blog/nourish-roots-importance-palliative-care-education -medical-school, March 25, 2020.
13. University of Rochester, "A New Way to Prepare Doctors for Difficult Conversations," July 15, 2021, www.rochester.edu/newscenter/virtual -patient-sophie-prepares-doctors-for-end-of-life-conversations -485392/.
14. Christine Cowgill, "Urgent Need for Better End-of-Life Training," *Today's Geriatric Medicine*, June 26, 2013.
15. Puri, *That Good Night*, 118.

16. Alistair Gardiner, "Most Physicians Feel They Lack This Type of Training," *MDLinx*, February 1, 2021.
17. The ABCDE approach (https://spcare.bmj.com/content/9/Suppl_1 /A15.1) and the SPIKES protocol (https://pubmed.ncbi.nlm.nih.gov /10964998/) may help physicians and nurses to practice more patient-centered end-of-life care.
18. Atul Gawande, "When Treating Patients, 'Our Core Goal Is to Enable Their Goals,' " *Healio*, June 1, 2019.
19. Rana L. A. Awdish, "A View from the Edge—Creating a Culture of Caring," *New England Journal of Medicine* 376, no. 1 (2017): 7–9.
20. Rana L. A. Awdish and Leonard L. Berry, "Making Time to Really Listen to Your Patients," *Harvard Business Review*, October 19, 2017.
21. Awdish, "A View from the Edge."
22. Center to Advance Palliative Care, "America's Care of Serious Illness."
23. Diane E. Meier et al., "A National Strategy for Palliative Care," *Health Affairs* 36, no. 7 (2017): 1266–73.
24. Meier et al., "A National Strategy."
25. National Coalition for Hospice and Palliative Care, "Palliative Care Guidelines," www.nationalcoalitionhpc.org/ncp.
26. Margot Sanger-Katz, "1,495 Americans Describe the Financial Reality of Being Really Sick," *New York Times*, October 17, 2018.
27. Center to Advance Palliative Care, "The Case for Community-Based Palliative Care," October 7, 2020.
28. Meier et al., "A National Strategy for Palliative Care."
29. Jim Parker, "Palliative Care Could Cut Health Care Costs by $103 Billion," *Hospice News*, April 4, 2019.
30. For more information on this program, visit www.vitaltalk.org.
31. VitalTalk, "About Us," www.vitaltalk.org/about-us.
32. Abbasi, "New Guidelines."
33. Sunita Puri, "Speaking from the Heart," End Well, https://endwellproject .org/speaking-from-the-heart.

Chapter 3. How We Want to Die
1. Ken Murray, "How Doctors Die: It's Not Like the Rest of Us, but It Should Be," *Zócalo Public Square*, November 30, 2011.
2. Emily Wilson, "How Doctors Die: Physicians Are Less Likely Than the General Population to Undergo Intense End-of-Life Treatments," Harvard Medical School, "News & Research," January 21, 2016.
3. Murray, "How Doctors Die."
4. Stanford School of Medicine, "Where Do Americans Die?," https:// palliative.stanford.edu/home-hospice-home-care-of-the-dying-patient /where-do-americans-die/#:~:text=Studies%20have%20shown %20that%20approximately,and%20only%2020%25%20at%20home.
5. Center to Advance Palliative Care, "Palliative Care Facts and Stats," https://media.capc.org/filer_public/68/bc/68bc93c7-14ad-4741-9830 -8691729618d0/capc_press-kit.pdf.

6. Center to Advance Palliative Care, "Palliative Care Facts and Stats."
7. Benzi M. Kluger et al., "Comparison of Integrated Outpatient Palliative Care with Standard Care in Patients with Parkinson Disease and Related Disorders: A Randomized Clinical Trial," *JAMA Neurology*, February 10, 2020.
8. Hebatalla Elhusseiny et al., "The Role of Palliative Care in Adult Moderate to Severe Traumatic Brain Injury," *Palliative Care: Open Access*, July 24, 2018.
9. Alicia Lasek and Peter Tanuseputro, "People with Dementia Receive Fewer Palliative Referrals Than Those with Cancer: Study," *Clinical Daily News*, March 5, 2021.
10. Ravi B. Parikh and Alexi A. Wright, "The Affordable Care Act and End-of-Life Care for Patients with Cancer," *Cancer Journal* 23, no. 3 (2018): 190–93.
11. Centers for Disease Control and Prevention, National Center for Chronic Disease Prevention and Health Promotion, "Division for Heart Disease and Stroke Prevention at a Glance," www.cdc.gov/chronicdisease /resources/publications/aag/heart-disease-stroke.htm.
12. Susan L. Hayes et al., "High-Need, High-Cost Patients: Who Are They and How Do They Use Health Care?," The Commonwealth Fund, August 29, 2016.
13. Kim Kuebler, "Policy and Practice Trends for Multiple Chronic Conditions," PowerPoint presentation, MPCA Spring Clinical Conference, April 2018; Wullianallur Raghupathi and Viju Raghupathi, "An Empirical Study of Chronic Diseases in the United States: A Visual Analytics Approach to Public Health," *International Journal of Environmental Research and Public Health* 15, no. 3 (2018): 431.
14. Hayes et al., "High-Need, High-Cost Patients."
15. Kim Kuebler, "Palliative Practices for Patients Living with Multiple Chronic Conditions," *Multiple Chronic Conditions* (blog), www.multiplechronicconditions.org.
16. Stacey Burling, "Study: Older Patients Avoid Life Expectancy Talk with Doctors," *Philadelphia Enquirer*, April 24, 2019.
17. Stephanie O'Neill, "Knowing How Doctors Die Can Change End-of-Life Discussions," NPR, *All Things Considered*, July 6, 2015.
18. Cynthia Rockwell, "Toward a Gentler Death: A Q&A with Katy Butler '71," *Wesleyan University Magazine*, May 10, 2018.
19. Sue Campbell, "Atul Gawande's 5 Questions to Ask at Life's End," *Next Avenue*, February 10, 2015.
20. Campbell, "Atul Gawande's 5 Questions."
21. Rebecca M. Saracino et al., "Geriatric Palliative Care: Meeting the Needs of a Growing Population," *Geriatric Nursing* 39, no. 2 (2018): 225–29.
22. Danielle D. DeCourcey et al., "Advance Care Planning and Parent-Reported End-of-Life Outcomes in Children, Adolescents, and Young

Adults with Complex Chronic Conditions," *Critical Care Medicine* 47, no. 1 (2019): 101–8.

23. Murray, "How Doctors Die."
24. Wilson, "How Doctors Die."
25. Wilson, "How Doctors Die."

Chapter 4. How to Get the Care You Want

1. Centers for Disease Control and Prevention, "Advance Care Planning: Ensuring Your Wishes Are Known and Honored If You Are Unable to Speak for Yourself," www.cdc.gov/aging/pdf/advanced-care-planning -critical-issue-brief.pdf.
2. Nichole Bazemore, "Here's Everything You Need to Know about the Patient's Bill of Rights," *Forbes*, March 21, 2016.
3. American Patient Rights Association, "AHA Patient's Bill of Rights," www.americanpatient.org/aha-patients-bill-of-rights.
4. American Patient Rights Association, "AHA Patient's Bill of Rights." For more information on the Patient's Bill of Rights, visit www.aha.org /other-resources/patient-care-partnership.
5. If you want more educational material on your condition, treatments, or procedures, you have the right to ask for it from a member of your team. Your doctor will not necessarily give it to you, but someone on your palliative care team will—typically either a nurse or a social worker, depending on what it pertains to. They might not have it on hand, but they will certainly have it in their medical records.
6. American Patient Rights Association, "AHA Patient's Bill of Rights."
7. Michelle Edelstein-Rutgers, "If Doctor Decides, Aggressive End-of-Life Care More Likely," *Futurity*, June 19, 2019.
8. Elizabeth Bailey, *The Patient's Checklist: 10 Simple Hospital Checklists to Keep You Safe, Sane, and Organized* (New York: Sterling, 2011).
9. GetPalliativeCare.org, "How to Get Palliative Care?" https://getpalliative care.org/howtoget.
10. Slidell Memorial Hospital, "7 Things to Do before, during, and after Your Hospital Stay," www.slidellmemorial.org/blog/7-things-to-do -before-during-and-after-your-hospital-stay.
11. Rachael Grannell, "7 Things You Should Absolutely Know before Going to the Hospital," *Huffington Post*, June 12, 2014.
12. Slidell Memorial Hospital, "7 Things to Do before, during, and after Your Hospital Stay."
13. HealthStream, "Recognizing Religious Beliefs in Healthcare," April 1, 2021, https://www.healthstream.com/resource/blog/recognizing -religious-beliefs-in-healthcare.
14. Esme Finlay et al., "Models of Outpatient Palliative Care Clinics for Patients with Cancer," *Journal of Oncology Practice* 15, no. 7 (2019): 187–93.

15. Jim Parker, "ACHC Launches Palliative Care Accreditation Program," *Hospice News*, April 19, 2021.

Chapter 5. How to Cope When Illness Changes Everything

1. HelpGuide, "Coping with a Life-Threatening Illness or Serious Health Event," www.helpguide.org/articles/grief/coping-with-a-life -threatening-illness.htm.
2. HelpGuide, "Coping with a Life-Threatening Illness."
3. Vitas Healthcare, "Complementary Therapies Increase Comfort, Well-Being of Hospice Patients," July 17, 2017.
4. AARP, "Can I Get Paid to Be a Caregiver for a Family Member?," July 1, 2021.
5. Meltem Dinleyici and Figen Şahin Dağlı, "Evaluation of Quality of Life of Healthy Siblings of Children with Chronic Disease," *Turkish Archives of Pediatrics* 53, no. 4 (2018): 205–13.
6. Elisabeth Kübler-Ross, *On Children and Death* (New York: Scribner, 1983), 68.
7. Afaf Girgis et al., "Physical, Psychosocial, Relationship, and Economic Burden of Caring for People with Cancer: A Review," *Journal of Oncology Practice*, December 9, 2012.
8. Elaine Y. L. Lung et al., "Informal Caregiving for People with Life-Limiting Illness: Exploring the Knowledge Gaps," *Journal of Palliative Care*, January 20, 2021.
9. Ann Brenoff, "No One Gives a Rat's Ass about Family Caregivers," *Huffington Post*, September 1, 2016.
10. Jill Slaboda et al., "A Study of Family Caregiver Burden and the Imperative of Practice Change to Address Family Caregivers' Unmet Needs," *HealthAffairs*, January 11, 2018.
11. Andrew Esch, "Coping Strategies and Resources for Family Caregivers," GetPalliativeCare.org, https://getpalliativecare.org/coping-strategies -and-resources-for-family-caregivers/?utm_source=email_caregivers &utm_medium=email_caregivers&utm_campaign=email_caregivers.

Chapter 6. Putting It All Together

1. Angelo E. Volandes, *The Conversation: A Revolutionary Plan for End-of-Life Care* (New York: Bloomsbury, 2015), book jacket.
2. Sunita Puri, "It's Time to Talk about Death and Coronavirus," *New York Times*, March 27, 2020.
3. Laura J. Morrison, "It's Time to Train All Doctors on How to Talk to Patients about End-of-Life Care," *Huffington Post*, June 15, 2016.
4. The Conversation Project, "About Us," https://theconversationproject .org/about.
5. Death Cafe, "What Is Death Cafe?," https://deathcafe.com/what.
6. Mary J. Isaacson and Mary E. Minton, "End-of-Life Communication:

Nurses Cocreating the Closing Composition with Patients and Families," *Advances in Nursing Science* 41, no. 1 (2018): 2–17.

7. National Hospice and Palliative Care Organization, "Conversations before the Crisis," 2017.
8. Priyanka Boghani, "Facing Mortality: How to Talk to Your Doctor," *Frontline*, February 10, 2015.
9. National Hospice and Palliative Care Organization, "Conversations before the Crisis."
10. National Hospice and Palliative Care Organization, "Conversations before the Crisis."
11. Boghani, "Facing Mortality."
12. Boghani, "Facing Mortality"; Cynthia F. Cramer, "To Live until You Die," *Clinical Journal of Oncology Nursing* 14, no. 1 (2010): 53–56.
13. Cramer, "To Live until You Die."
14. Jo Cavallo, "Advance Care Planning: Ensuring Patients' End-of-Life Wishes Are Honored," *ASCO Post*, July 25, 2017.
15. For more information, visit https://fivewishes.org.
16. VJ Periyakoil, "Who Is the Designated Driver, or Proxy, for Your Health Decisions?," *Scope 10K*, September 25, 2018.
17. Bruce Horovitz, "Pandemic Isn't Spurring Older Adults to Discuss, Record Advance Health Care Wishes," *AARP*, April 6, 2021.
18. POLST forms are available only in some states. You can find out if your state is included and learn more at www.polst.org. If you would like to have a POLST form, talk to your health care team about your wishes.
19. New England Donor Services, https://neds.org/register-now. Each state has different requirements for organ donation; visit www.organdonor.gov for more information. Many donors may wish to register through both Donate Life and their state's Department of Motor Vehicles. You can change your mind about donation; you will need to notify either your state's Department of Motor Vehicles or Donate Life America by going to www.registerme.org.
20. Carolyn Crist, "CPR Survival Rates Are Lower Than Most People Think," Reuters, February 23, 2018.
21. Paula Span, "The Patients Were Saved. That's Why the Families Are Suing," *New York Times*, April 10, 2017.
22. Amy Berman, "A Nurse with Fatal Breast Cancer Says End-of-Life Discussions Save Her Life," *Washington Post*, September 28, 2015.
23. Amy Berman, "Narrative Matters, the Next Chapter: Amy Berman Reflects on 'Living Life in My Own Way,'" *Health Affairs*, May 22, 2014.

Chapter 7. Spirituality and Well-Being

1. Christina Puchalski, "Spirituality as an Essential Domain of Palliative Care: Caring for the Whole Person," *Progress in Palliative Care* 20, no. 2 (2013): 63–65.

2. Puchalski, "Spirituality as an Essential Domain."
3. Puchalski, "Spirituality as an Essential Domain."
4. Adam Brady, "Religion and Spirituality: The Difference between Them," *Chopra.com*, August 4, 2020.
5. Fetzer Institute, "What Does Spirituality Mean to Us? A Study of Spirituality in the United States," September 2020.
6. Fetzer, "What Does Spirituality Mean to Us?"
7. Gary McCord et al., "Discussing Spirituality with Patients: A Rational and Ethical Approach," *Annals of Family Medicine* 2, no. 4 (2004): 356–61.
8. Robin Bennett Kanarek, "Spiritual Distress Manifested in a Teenager after a Stem Cell Transplant," *Journal of Pain and Symptom Management* 60, no. 1 (2020): 176–78.
9. Puchalski, "Spirituality as an Essential Domain."
10. CaringInfo, "It's about How You LIVE in Faith," http://il-hpco.org/wp-content/uploads/2016/03/Faith_Community_Outreach_Guide.pdf; Duke Institute on Care at the End of Life, "Offering Spiritual Support for Family or Friends."
11. Tracy A. Balboni et al., "Religiousness and Spiritual Support among Advanced Cancer Patients and Associations with End-of-Life Treatment Preferences and Quality of Life," *Journal of Clinical Oncology* 25, no. 5 (2007): 555–60.
12. McCord et al., "Discussing Spirituality with Patients."
13. Rebekah Schmidt, "The Role of Chaplaincy in Caring for the Seriously Ill," *Palliative Care Network of Wisconsin*, December 2017.
14. The Joint Commission, "Part 1. Body, Mind, Spirit: Hospital Chaplains Contribute to Patient Satisfaction and Well-Being," *The Source* 16, no. 1 (2018): 11.
15. Tyler J. VanderWeele, Tracy A. Balboni, and Howard K. Koh, "Health and Spirituality," *Journal of the American Medical Association* 318, no. 6 (2017): 519–20.
16. Jim Kling, "Spirituality an Important Component of Patient Care: An Expert Interview with Christina M. Puchalski, MD," *Medscape*, March 2, 2011.
17. Center to Advance Palliative Care, "Specialty Palliative Care Certification," www.capc.org/jobs/palliative-care-certification.
18. Patrice Richardson, "Spirituality, Religion, and Palliative Care," *Annals of Palliative Medicine* 3, no. 3 (2014): 150–59.
19. Marc Haufe et al., "How Can Existential or Spiritual Strengths Be Fostered in Palliative Care? An Interpretative Synthesis of Recent Literature," *BMJ Supportive and Palliative Care*, September 14, 2020.
20. Haufe et al., "How Can Existential or Spiritual Strengths Be Fostered?"
21. Viktor Frankl, *Man's Search for Meaning* (Boston: Beacon Press, 1959).

22. Jewish Broadcasting Service, "L'Chayim: Robin Kanarek (Transcending Loss)," a conversation with Rabbi Mark Golub, May 23, 2019, https://www.youtube.com/watch?v=LDHFq5vfN10.

23. Cynthia F. Cramer, "To Live Until You Die," *Clinical Journal of Oncology Nursing* 14, no. 1 (2010): 53–56.

24. Haufe et al., "How Can Existential or Spiritual Strengths Be Fostered?"

Chapter 8. Grief

1. Georgena Eggleston, "Grief Brain Equals Brain Fog," *Beyond Your Loss*, January 27, 2019.

2. Stephanie O'Neill, "Grief for Beginners: 5 Things to Know about Processing Loss," NPR, May 14, 2020.

3. David Kessler and Elisabeth Kübler-Ross, *Finding Meaning: The Sixth Stage of Grief* (New York: Scribner, 2019), 29.

4. Carolyn Jaffe and Carol H. Ehrlich, "Only God Knows When," in *All Kinds of Love: Experiencing Hospice* (Amityville, NY: Baywood Publishing, 1997).

5. Cleveland Clinic, "Grief: What's Normal, What's Not—and 13 Tips to Get through It," July 27, 2018.

6. Paul J. Moon, "Grief and Palliative Care: Mutuality," *Palliative Care: Research and Treatment* 7 (2013): 19–24.

7. O'Neill, "Grief for Beginners."

Chapter 9. Making Palliative Care Mainstream

1. Jim Parker, "New Senate Caucus to Focus on Palliative Care," *Hospice News*, July 31, 2019; Jim Parker, "House Approves Hospice Education Act," *Hospice News*, October 28, 2019.

2. National Hospice and Palliative Care Organization, www.nhpco.org/advocacy.

3. Trish Riley and Kitty Purington, "States Chart a Policy Path to Improve Palliative Care Services across the Care Continuum," *Health Affairs*, August 13, 2019.

4. Cambia Palliative Care Center of Excellence, https://depts.washington.edu/pallcntr/index.html.

5. Peggy Maguire and Steven Z. Pantilat, "Foundation Addresses Critical Need for Palliative Care Workforce and Leadership Development," *Health Affairs*, July 13, 2017.

6. Robert Wood Johnson Foundation, "Our Guiding Principles," https://www.rwjf.org/en/about-rwjf/our-guiding-principles.html.

7. Ira Byock et al., "Promoting Excellence in End-of-Life Care," abstract, *PubMed*, https://pubmed.ncbi.nlm.nih.gov/16430353.

8. 2020NurseandMidwife, "Nurses by the Numbers," https://2020nurseandmidwife.org/nurses-by-the-numbers.

9. Betty Ferrell et al., "CARES: AACN's New Competencies and Recommendations for Educating Undergraduate Nursing Students to Improve Palliative Care," *Journal of Professional Nursing*, September/October 2016.

10. Ellen Rice Tichich, "Improving Palliative Care through Education," *Oncology Nursing News*, January/February 2019.

11. Ferrell et al., "CARES: AACN's New Competencies."

12. Tammy Neiman, "Acute Care Nurses' Experiences of Basic Palliative Care," *Journal of Hospice & Palliative Nursing*, January 25, 2020.

13. Maguire and Pantilat, "Foundation Addresses Critical Need."

14. Robin Kanarek and Vikky Riley, "The Parent's Perspective of Teenage Cancer," in T. O. B. Eden et al., eds., *Cancer and the Adolescent*, 2nd ed. (Oxford: Blackwell Publishing, 2005), 214–27.

15. Constance Dahlin and Patrick Coyne, "The Palliative APRN Leader," *Annals of Palliative Medicine* 8, no. 1 (2019): S30–S38.

16. Constance Dahlin et al., "Palliative Care Leadership," *Journal of Palliative Care* 34, no. 1 (2019): 21–28.

17. Palliative Care Leadership Centers, "How PCLC Works," www.capc.org /palliative-care-leadership-centers/how-pclc-works.

18. Dahlin et al., "Palliative Care Leadership."

19. Jane Phillips et al. "Nursing and Palliative Care," in Roderick Duncan MacLeod and Lieve Van den Block, eds., *Textbook of Palliative Care* (Basel, Switzerland: Springer, 2018), 1–16.

20. Juliette Cubanski et al., "Medicare Spending at the End of Life: A Snapshot of Beneficiaries Who Died in 2014 and the Cost of Their Care," *KFF*, www.kff.org/medicare/issue-brief/medicare-spending-at-the -end-of-life.

21. Center to Advance Palliative Care, "Trinity Health System: Transforming the Care of People Living with Serious Illness Using CAPC Membership," www.capc.org/membership/member-impact-stories/trinity -health-system-transforming-care-people-living-serious-illness-using -capc-membership.

22. Meg Bryant, "High Costs Give Palliative Care Increased Industry Interest," *Healthcare Dive*, February 15, 2017.

23. Bryant, "High Costs Give Palliative Care."

24. Catherine Riffin et al., "Identifying Key Priorities for Future Palliative Care Research Using an Innovative Analytic Approach," *American Journal of Public Health* 105, no. 1 (2015): e15–e21.

25. Riffin et al., "Identifying Key Priorities."

26. Mihir Kamdar, Joshua Lakin, and Haipeng Zhang, "Artificial Intelligence, Machine Learning, and Digital Therapeutics in Palliative Care and Hospice: The Future of Compassionate Care or Rise of the Robots?" *Journal of Pain and Symptom Management* 59, no. 2 (2020): 434–45.

27. Sheila Payne, Mark Tanner, and Sean Hughes, "Digitisation and the Patient-Professional Relationship in Palliative Care," *Journal of Palliative Care*, April 7, 2020.

28. Payne, Tanner, and Hughes, "Digitisation and the Patient-Professional Relationship."

Epilogue. David's Legacy

1. Robin Bennett Kanarek, "Life-Threatening Illness and a Mother's Emotional Journey: Lessons in Care," *Journal of Palliative Medicine* 20, no. 6 (2017): 684–86.

Index

Call for Action: Nurses Lead and
Transform Palliative Care, 158–59
Cambia Health Foundation, 159,
160–61; Palliative Care Center of
Excellence, 156
cancer care: adolescents, children,
young adults, 1–6, 50, 143,
161–62, 171–72; concurrent with
palliative care, 17, 25–26, 27–28,
49, 50, 52; pain management, 19
cardiopulmonary resuscitation
(CPR), 109–10, 112, 113
CARES Act, 53, 99
Carter, Rosalyn, 98
Centers for Disease Control and
Prevention (CDC), 52, 67
Center to Advance Palliative Care
(CAPC), 10–11, 22, 35–36,
40–41, 42–43, 49, 157, 162, 163,
165; Palliative Care Leadership
Centers, 163
Centre for Palliative Care,
Melbourne University, 24
chaplains, 12, 37, 43, 45, 79, 125, 126,
129–30; palliative care training
and certification, 41–42, 130–31,
136–37, 156, 170
Chaturvedi, Aditi, "Complemen-
tary and Alternative Medicine in
Cancer Pain Management"
(article), 19–20
chemotherapy, 14–15, 16, 27, 32, 68,
97, 115, 116, 133
children. *See* adolescents, children,
young adults
chronic illnesses, 59; multiple, 53–55,
56
Churchill, Winston, 8, 141
City of Hope, 16–17
Cleveland Clinic, 78, 145–46
cognitive behavioral therapy, 19
College of Pastoral Supervision and
Psychotherapy, 130–31
comfort care. *See* palliative care
Commonwealth Fund, 42

communication, patient-family:
end-of-life care, 103, 106–9,
114–15, 127; as spiritual support,
125–27
communication, patient–health
care provider, 43; COMFORT
model, 105–6; communication
skills for, 43–44, 106–7, 170;
death and dying, 4–5, 45, 48,
55–57, 61–62, 64, 104–6, 118;
empathy in, 38–40, 62; end-of-
life care, 37, 55–59, 102–3, 108–9,
128; palliative care, 4–5, 7–8,
27–28, 32–33, 36, 37, 74–75,
115–16; physician's avoidance,
68; questions to ask, 73–75, 78
communication with and within
medical care teams, 43–45, 114
communication within families:
end-of-life care, 114–15; during
grieving process, 144
Community Health Accreditation
Partner, 41–42
complementary and alternative
medicine, 19–20, 87, 133
Comskil program, 44
constipation, 15, 16, 17–18, 50
Conversation Project, 105, 108
Cooney, Gail Austin, 6–7
coping skills, 83–87, 92–93, 94,
121–22; for grief, 142–50
cortisol, 138–39
Cowgill, Christine and Robert,
Soul Service (book), 37–38
Cramer, Cynthia, 135
curative treatment: concurrent with
palliative care, 12, 16, 18, 24, 33,
35, 49, 50, 70; physicians' focus
on, 32–34, 36, 130, 169

Dahlin, Constance, 162–63
Daniel, Terri, 150
death and dying, 56, 58, 85; at
home, 47–48, 52, 64, 65, 102; in
hospitals, 47–48, 52, 67–68, 72,

Index • 205

Kaiser Permanente Colorado, Supportive Care Solutions, 34
Kanarek, David Bennett, 1–6, 8–9, 28–31, 90, 91, 92–93, 118, 119, 122–23, 124, 127, 128, 134; acute lymphocytic leukemia, 1–6, 32–33, 60–63, 73; death, 138–40, 142–43, 145, 150, 170; legacy, 9, 122, 143, 148, 163, 169–72; sense of humor, 96–98, 148–49; stem cell transplant, 3–4, 28–29, 32–33, 62, 76, 83, 88–89, 92, 94, 118, 122
Kanarek, Joe, 1, 3, 29, 30, 44, 61–63, 83, 88–89, 92, 93, 95, 96–97, 122, 128, 134, 137, 140, 143, 148
Kanarek, Robin Bennett, 137; "Life-Threatening Illness and a Mother's Emotional Journey" (essay), 170–71; "Palliative Care Isn't Just for the Dying" (article), 6–7; "The Parent's Perspective of Teenage Cancer" (book chapter) 161–62, "Spiritual Distress Manifested in a Teenager after a Stem Cell Transplant" (essay), 123
Kanarek, Sarah, 3, 29–30, 83, 88–89, 90, 93, 94, 122–23, 132, 143, 144
Kanarek Center for Palliative Care, 122, 163, 171
Kanarek Family Foundation, 9, 148, 171
Kessler, David, *Finding Meaning* (book), 141–42
kidney (renal) disease/failure, 22, 49, 50, 52–53, 55, 56–57, 58–59
Kübler-Ross, Elisabeth, 122, 138, 140; *Finding Meaning* (book), 141–42; *On Children and Death* (book), 89–90

leadership in palliative care, 153, 156, 159, 161–64, 171
legislation affecting palliative care, 52–53, 100, 152, 153–55
life expectancy, 25–28, 55–56
life-prolonging treatment, 16, 24, 63, 67–68, 104, 113; aggressive approach, 9, 48, 60, 63, 67, 72, 102, 108, 113. *See also* advance directives; living wills
limited medical care, 104
liver disease, 35, 39, 53
living wills, 70, 75, 76, 77–78, 110
loneliness, 146
loss, 30, 38, 118, 132, 133; of self, 85, 118. *See also* grief
lung disease, 22, 50, 53

Maguire, Peggy, 160–61
malpractice litigation, 64
marital issues, 93–96
Massachusetts, palliative care initiatives in, 26, 102, 106
Massachusetts General Hospital, 25, 26, 102, 106
mastectomy, 27, 115
meaningful life, 7, 11, 34, 46, 48–49, 74, 84, 108, 118, 130
Medicaid, 87–88, 155
medical care teams, 36; communication issues, 43–45, 61, 73
medical errors, 73
Medical Orders for Life-Sustaining Treatment (MOLST) form, 113
medical specialties and specialists, 36, 49–50; palliative care specialty, 10–11, 13, 22, 36, 153
medical terminology, 78–79
Medicare, 52, 53, 56
medications: allergies and side effects, 76, 77–78; for pain management, 18–19, 20, 23; polypharmacy, 54
Meier, Diane, 22–23, 40–41, 162, 165–66
Memorial Sloan Kettering Cancer Center, 19, 44, 61, 94, 132, 161–62, 171

memories of deceased loved ones, 148–49, 150
Mental Health Parity Act (MHPA), 153–54
Merino, Jim, 78
mind-body-spirit connection, 84–85, 116
Moon, Paul J., 149
multiple sclerosis, 50
Murphy, Phil, 154
Murray, Kenneth, "How Doctors Die" (essay), 47–48, 60

narcotics/opioids, 18–19, 20, 23
National Academy for State Health Policy, 155
National Association of Social Workers, 131
National Comprehensive Cancer Network (NCCN), 17
National Consensus Project for Quality Palliative Care, 41, 160
National Council on Aging, 53
National Hospice and Palliative Care Organization, 24, 106, 125–26, 131, 163
National Institute on Aging, 99
National Institutes of Health, 44, 53
nausea/vomiting, 15, 17–18, 20, 50
New York Presbyterian Hospital, 61
Nuland, Sherwin, *How We Die* (book), 59
nurses: communication role, 43, 44; palliative care certification, 41–42, 131; palliative care education, 37–38, 152, 156, 157–60, 171; palliative care leadership role, 153, 159, 161–64, 171; as palliative care team members, 12
nursing homes, 18, 36, 48, 164

Obama, Barack, 52, 68–69
occupational therapy/therapists, 12, 87, 132, 133
older adults: and advance care

planning, 55–59; baby boomers, 9, 35, 49; and multiple chronic conditions, 54, 55–56; and telehealth access, 52–53
oncologists, 2, 14–15, 16, 22, 27–28, 115. *See also* cancer care
oncology, pediatric, 1–6, 50, 59–63, 72, 143, 161–62, 171–72. *See also* cancer care
oncology team, 17
organ failure, 51
organ transplants, 49–50, 62, 112; donation registration, 112
OSF HealthCare, 165–66

pain: fear of, 20, 109; tolerance levels, 20
pain management, 7, 13, 16, 23, 50, 74–75, 109, 110, 130; at home, 65; after hospital discharge, 80; therapeutic options, 18–20, 23; total pain concept, 16–18, 119
palliative care, 59, 65–66; accessibility and utilization, 152–68; awareness of, 55, 155, 167–68; benefits to caregivers, 50, 99–100; certification and accreditation programs, 41–42; clinical practice guidelines, 17, 41, 165; definitions, 10–11, 13, 18, 24, 34, 104; early, 24–25, 27–28, 115–16; future priorities for, 166–67; goals, 7, 10–11, 12, 23, 24, 46, 48–49, 84; initiation of, 12, 16, 17, 18, 21, 25, 26; late-stage, 25, 26; mid-stage, 24; misconceptions/misunderstandings about, 22–24, 26, 34, 55, 117; for noncancer conditions, 49–51; outpatient, 80–81; physicians' failure to offer, 4, 8–9, 22–23, 28, 36; relation to hospice care, 6–7, 8, 14, 18, 22, 25, 155; requests for, 15, 16, 23, 26, 33, 45, 68, 70, 74; research and innovations, 166–67;

About the Author

Robin Kanarek has worked as a registered nurse since 1980 in a multitude of nursing specialties focusing on chronic medical conditions, including cardiac rehabilitation, diabetes, stroke, and spinal cord injuries. Nothing prepared her, however, for the most emotionally charged experience she would ever face: her son's diagnosis with leukemia at the age of ten. She and her husband worked together as one to get David well. Unfortunately, after five years, he succumbed to the complications of the disease. It took Robin and her family many years to find a way to live with their loss. She learned over time that she had a powerful voice as a nurse, mother, and advocate for palliative care. Robin has spoken about her family and her son's experience at international and national conferences, has been published in numerous prestigious medical and nursing journals, and has worked with the top leaders and institutions in health care. She is the founder and president of the Kanarek Family Foundation, whose mission is to improve the quality of life for those affected by cancer and other serious, life-threatening conditions through the promotion, education, and integration of palliative and supportive care into all areas of health care. Proceeds from this book will be used to continue to improve palliative care and to honor David's short but remarkable life.

You can find Robin on her websites at RobinKanarek.com or KanarekFamilyFoundation.org, on Twitter at @rbennk, or on LinkedIn at linkedin.com/in/robin-bennett-kanarek-3605a9167.

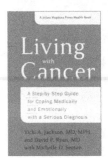 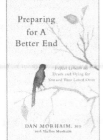 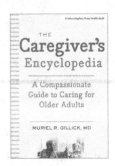 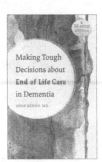

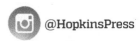
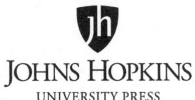